Move Right. Live Right.

What the mind believes capable, becomes capable: Strategies to move towards a better you

Daniel Cooper

To Sarah, thank you for always believing, supporting and encouraging me.

Contents

Foreword

L et me introduce myself.

My name is Daniel Cooper. I am a clinical exercise physiologist, personal trainer and business owner of 'Move Right EP'. I have worked with a range of people from different backgrounds, ages and medical histories. I am a constant learner, I strive to understand, implement and create programmes to change your movement so you can live the life you want to.

Throughout my life I have been met with injury, questions I had no way of answering at the time. I longed for a book like this to guide me and educate me around the crazy intricacies of the physiological, psychological and emotional aspects that present when working with people.

This is a book from me to you. I want to share my knowledge and experiences through both anecdotal and evidence-based research and implications to allow you to understand your body, how you can improve it and how to take independence with your training. This will also equip you with the foundations towards helping others! Not just a 'self-help' book but rather a help book, you or the people you are working with!

Within this book will entail evidence, my own understanding of it and some ambiguity. I want this book to make you question yourself and reflect within.

This book will serve as a guide, a tool for you to keep adherent, accountable and structured on your endeavour to improve your body, your mind and your life.

No matter who you are, this reading will be of use to you.

Are you new to training? Prepare to learn!

Spent a fair share of your time in the gym? You will take something away from this, I guarantee!

Qualified practitioner? You will improve your quality of care for your patients!

The information within this book should be referred to throughout various stages of your life, you will come back to the chapters with new knowledge and this will alter your perspectives of what you read over and over.

1

Compression & Expansion

"Breathing, according to me, corresponds to taking charge of one's own life." - Luce Irigaray

T he universe is currently in a constant state of expansion.

We know that everything that exists within our known universe was once condensed or compressed before a massive reaction i.e., the Big Bang, which led to the start of the world we know today.

Everything since the beginning of this universe abides by various laws, some known and I'm sure a hell of a lot remain unknown; these laws govern you, me and everything that is.

Think of breathing like the start of your own personal universe. You inspire or breathe, allowing air to enter the lungs. That air circulates and mixes with blood from your heart before being pushed around to the surrounding organs, tissues and muscles quickly and efficiently. You supply your body with life. Nutrients and oxygen permeate every cell and allow growth.

Then you breathe out, you expire, and the used or deoxygenated air now leaves the lungs and goes back out into the atmosphere, and the cycle renews again, and again and again.

Keep it simple. You take a breath in; you expand and give your body nutrients. You take a breath out; you compress and get rid of waste throughout the body.

What's the fuss with all this breathing talk? You buy a self-help book expecting to learn about essential training and health concepts, and you've just read a spiel about breathing?

What the hell, you're thinking.

Please, let me explain why this is such an important concept to movement, training and your life.

Breathing is integral to living. As you're hopefully aware by now, if you don't breathe you will die.

We take approximately 23,000 breathes per day, every day.

Breathing is no different to anything else we do, whether it's writing, driving or exercising: there is a technique that creates an optimal pattern, allowing us to take fully efficient and effective breaths. If this optimal pattern is not achieved, then our body in its entirety will change. A common compensation arises in the form of movement – our range of motion can decrease, restricting you from touching your toes or reaching your arms above your head.

Many aspects influence our breathing. Our response to situations can change – our breathing reacts to anxiety and stress, either accelerating or decelerating, which can alter our mood.

This change in frequency often leads to subtle alterations until the point that you can no longer move properly. This may lead you to see a practitioner like myself.

A lack of movement can influence the body's tissues and, due to the relationship between breathing and the nervous system, painful symptoms can also arise. This may lead to debilitation, an inability to carry out simple daily activities like carrying your shopping inside or unloading the dishwasher.

Will this happen to everyone with a movement deficiency? Not necessarily, but given enough time and compensations in movement, pain often creeps up on us.

WHAT FACTORS INFLUENCE OUR BREATHING?

Well, simply put, life.

- We get stressed

- We get injured

- We get excited

- We aren't conscious of how we breathe in particular circumstances

- Posture

- We favour a particular pattern more than others

- Sport

- Work

WHAT DOES CHANGING OUR BREATHING RATE DO TO US?

A range of physiological processes are influenced by the rate of our breath.

Before we delve into this, we should first understand our nervous system.

Enter ... the autonomic nervous system (ANS). This in-built system is within you, me and every other human being; all animals, in fact. The ANS is controlled by an area of your brain called the hypothalamus – a key regulator of multiple parts of your body, such as the cardiovascular system, respiratory system, reflexes and other processes such as coughing and sneezing.

Have you ever thought to yourself about breathing? The fact that we breathe approximately 23,000 breathes a day and barely think about breathing should blow you away. This is the result of your ANS, working tirelessly to keep you alive. Our breathing can bias us towards the sympathetic or the parasympathetic – we can use this to our advantage, but the fact that breathing is largely autonomous can also be disadvantageous.

Now, the ANS can be further broken down into two subgroups or systems.

These are:

The sympathetic nervous system (SNS) – fight or flight.

The parasympathetic nervous system (PNS) – rest and digest.

The PNS, or the catchy term 'rest and digest', controls a host of functions around your muscle tone, specifically reducing it. Inducing relaxation and decreasing your overall energy expenditure, it is often known as an inhibitory pathway within your body. This is what we tap into when we practice relaxation techniques – yoga, meditation, mindfulness, tai chi, deep breathing, grounding. These all work on the predictable pattern that occurs within our brain as a result of slowing down our breath, biasing us towards our PNS.

Another way to think about this is after a stressful day. You know, you sit down on your lounge and take a deep breath out or sigh. This is you compressing your body, allowing everything to be expelled, relaxing it from the previous stresses.

Our second system, the SNS, is often associated with the phrase 'fight or flight', meaning we use this to either amp up our energy and fight or to run away.

Our brain is unable to perceive our external environment visually; instead, it receives feedback from a range of different sources or senses – sight, sound, touch, taste and smell. Meaning your brain recognises a stressful situation but cannot see it.

What does this look like? you ask.

You may be sitting behind your desk with work piling up around you, making you feel like you will be stuck in the office for a lifetime, or you may literally be running from a lion in the barren lands of Africa after a trip went horribly wrong (I know, I like to exaggerate with extreme examples).

In each case your SNS will be called upon. You will increase your muscle tone, narrow your focus, increase your energy expenditure by changing the pace of your breathing i.e., your heart pumps faster to get those much-needed nutrients and oxygen to your organs and muscles so you can fight or run.

Can you see how this situation can be beneficial but also determinantal?

On the one hand, we are sitting behind a desk, on the other fighting for our lives, yet we have the same response. If we live in this state for a chronic period, that is when we wreak havoc on our bodies. Letting this go unchecked will affect you physiologically in a multitude of ways.

Now, inhalation is classified as an SNS-based process while exhalation is the opposite, focusing more on the PNS processes. We need both of these states for functioning; one is not more important than the other. It is when we are biased towards a particular one over a long period of time that we adapt our way of living and make this our normality.

Do you see the problem in living in a perpetual state of stress?

Inhalation is an element of the expansion movement strategy, and exhalation is an element of the compression movement strategy. Both inhalation and exhalation can be attributed to everyday bodily functions. These two strategies, when viewed from either movement of joints or a biomechanical point of view, display opposite motions.

Bear with me.

The expansion movement strategy may be viewed in terms of flexion, abduction, external rotation, supination and plantar flexion. The element is associated with eccentric or lengthening of a muscle. Think of turning your palms forward and straightening your arm.

The compression movement strategy may be viewed in complete contrast. It involves actions of extension, adduction, internal rotation, pronation and dorsiflexion of the joints. As you may have guessed, the compression strategy is associated with the concentric or shorting of a muscle. Think of this like turning your palm towards the floor and bending your arm towards your face.

We will delve into this later, but for now, this basic understanding should stay in the back of your mind.

In an ideal skeleton, we can achieve both the expansion and compression of a joint. Movement limitations will more than likely occur due to breathing. The breathing cycle cannot be understated when trying to make noticeable change with movement.

Some questions to consider when looking to change your movement:

- Have you ever tried stretching to improve your flexibility or mobility?

- Have you noticed how you breathe?

- Do you hold your breath or breathe fluently?

This is, again, a nervous system response. Through the holding of our breath, we are in a state of inhalation; upregulating our sympathetic activation of 'for flight'. If we have not exhaled, we have not tapped into our parasympathetic state. This is an error commonly seen when people are being told how to stretch.

A classic example is giving someone a stretch and telling them to hold it for 30 seconds, only for them to rush through the counting, hold their breath and strain themselves. Their face ends up looking similar to a tomato. Do you think this is productive?

To make meaningful steps in accessing desired ranges of motion, fluent movement and a healthier way of living, we need to teach people how to move into new joint positions while regulating their breathing in a conscious, controlled manner. This is how we create lasting movement change. Rather than giving people a timeframe to hold a stretch, try asking them to hold a stretch for a number of breaths, say between five and 10 deep ones. You will be surprised by how much easier these positions become when the position of the bones is coordinated with breathing.

It is evident that our breath can change a multitude of physiological processes within our body, ranging from cortisol levels (stress), blood flow mechanics (vasoconstriction and dilation), heart rate variability, blood pressure control and more.[1,2]

The effects of breathing have barely been uncovered and recognised within the world of modern medicine. However, research exists promoting the influence that it can have. Eastern cultures, for example, Tibetan monks, have controlled their breath for millennia, creating amazing feats of regulating their core body temperature even within extreme environments such as the icy heartlands of Mt Everest.

Now, let's get you up and moving. Grab a camera, and set it up so you can see your thorax or midsection.

TEST YOURSELF – ARE YOU COMPRESSED OR EXPANDED?

What you should be looking for is expansion (like a balloon inflating) around your rib cage – front, side and back during the inhalation – as well as a healthy compression of the ribcage coming back in after the exhalation.

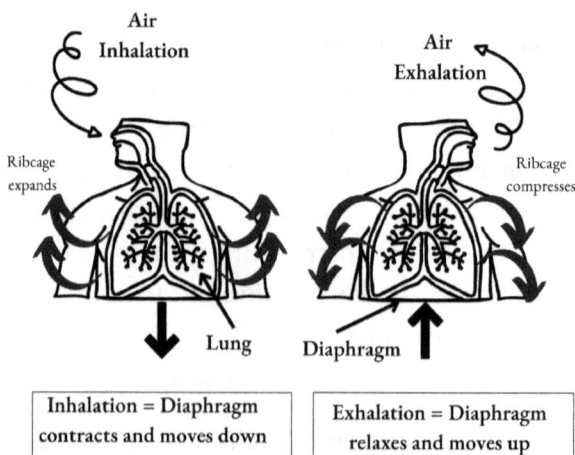

Air
Inhalation

Air
Exhalation

Ribcage
expands

Ribcage
compresses

Lung   Diaphragm

Inhalation = Diaphragm contracts and moves down	Exhalation = Diaphragm relaxes and moves up

Figure 1.1

Next, let's pay attention to how long you are breathing. For the purpose of this test, I want you to pay attention to how long you are exhaling.

Is this happening? Great, you're alive!

Now actually think about if you have an even ratio for breathing in vs. breathing out.

Look at your stomach, your chest; what is moving in and out?

Are you elevating your ribcage, depressing your ribcage or keeping your ribcage normal as you can see in Figure 1.2?

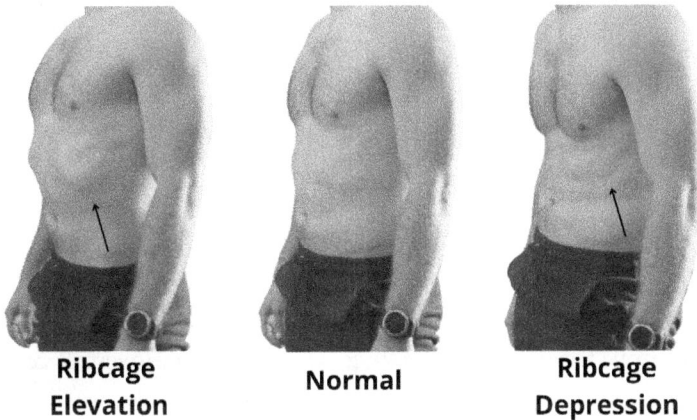

Ribcage Elevation   **Normal**   **Ribcage Depression**

Figure 1.2

The centre image is ideal.

The ribcage elevation is a sign that you are expanded in the front of your ribcage, and compressed at the back. With the ribcage depression, you are compressing the front of your ribcage and expanding at the back. Again, there's a time and place, but during rest, we should have a decent expansion around the whole ribcage like our image in the centre.

If this compression of the posterior or back side of your rib cage occurs, chances are you will exhibit a very shallow exhale and an anterior pelvic tilt; the drill below will enable you to allow the ribs to descend down and in (like they should).

A USEFUL DRILL – JOINT STACKING

What we are looking for is something called 'stacking' – simply put, if we start at your head and work our way down, we want each major bone stacked on top of one another in a line. If we look at the image below, we can see a centred rib cage on the left, where my shoulder girdle (the centre of my shoulder) and ribcage sit directly over my hips (pelvis), which sits directly over the knee, which sits directly over the ankle – almost like a straight line through the centre of our joints.

In the image on the right, compensation is apparent in the position I alluded to earlier. In this position, we have a change in the centre of gravity expansion on the front of the body and compression on the back of the body. The ribs are flaring upwards, causing the bones below to become 'unstacked' e.g., the hips move forward past the knee, and the knee moves off centre with the ankle. To prevent us from falling forward now that our hips are past our knees, we will instinctively lean backwards with our torso, leading to the image you can see in Figure 1.3.

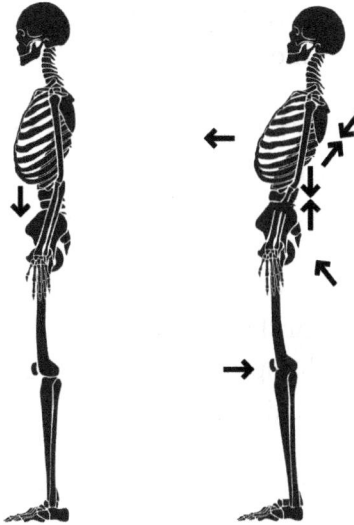

Figure 1.3

WHY IS IT IMPORTANT TO KEEP A STACKED POSITION?

Well, as our bones shift and move, our muscles react by short-ening and lengthening. Our muscles and joints each have an optimal position in which they can do what they are meant to do (make us move). If the bones move out of position, so do the muscles, leading to compensation which may present as muscle tightness or pain, lack of energy and so on.

This is known as the length-tension relationship – much more on this in Chapter 3.

SO ... HOW DO WE RESET OUR BREATHING?

TRY THE STEPS BELOW:

1. Lay on your back, and place one hand on your stomach, and the other on your chest. What we would ideally

see is the hand on your chest rising and falling as you breathe in and out.

2. Take a deep breath in through your nose. Now, focus on the exhale: try breathing out of your mouth; imagine fogging up glass with your breath.

3. While doing this, try and push past the point that you would normally breathe out. Generally, research suggests that the optimal time for a breath is 5.5 seconds in and 5.5 seconds out.

What you should feel is your rib cage compress down and in, and your stomach muscles switch on.

Focusing on a quality exhalation (outward breath) allows your bones to drop down (compress).

Now, the above steps are focused on compression; suited more for someone who lives in an expanded state. We do not need to breathe (trying to fog up glass forcefully) with each exhalation; this technique is more of a resetting, giving us joint and body awareness (proprioception) and allowing us to find our centre. People will often start in a state of imbalance, relying on compression or expansion for too long and becoming fixated in this posture. Use this tool as a reset and work from there.

This is a conscious effort at first. It will feel strange if you have not been breathing in this particular way. There is an element of skill involved, and it should not be rushed.

To begin with this will take a lot of focus and attention, so best to do it while you are in a quiet place and not distracted – so performing this while driving is off the table! Sorry to all your multi-taskers out there.

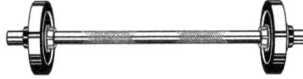

Let's recap

1. Breathing affects our autonomic system (sympathetic and parasympathetic).

2. Sympathetic is associated with inhalation (fight or flight) and parasympathetic is associated with exhalation (rest and digest).

3. People tend to breathe poorly more often than not due to their lifestyle and various other factors.

4. If we breathe poorly, we change our physiology – movement, stress, mood and a multitude of other physiological processes.

5. If we wish to see meaningful movement change, we need to encourage breathing in a conscious, controlled manner.

6. We need to expand our ribcage (like a balloon) 360 degrees with each inhalation.

7. We need to compress our ribcage with each exhalation.

8. We should be 'stacked' when undertaking the majority of activities, meaning our bones are in alignment (think hips over knees in a standing position).

9. The optimal breath is 5.5 seconds in, 5.5 seconds out – this equates to 5.5 breaths per minute.

2

Repeat After Me -- You Aren't a Terminator

"The primary and most beautiful of nature's qualities is motion" -Marquis De Sade

The body has 3 basic goals:

These are:

1. Breathe

2. Stay Alive/Upright

3. Move / Procreate

Not one of these is hunting and killing humans, like a terminator from James Cameron's movies. If you watch those movies, you will see a robot, built like a human. Aside from missing a conscience, they also miss quality movement. Terminators are stiff, hard and rigid. Don't be a terminator.

As humans or bipedal organisms, we have developed a structural adaptation to enable us to move forward through walking and running via an efficient mechanical process. The biomechanics of human locomotion is one we have measured, deconstructed and utilised to understand, improve upon and repair movement across healthy and unhealthy individuals.

With our training, each and every exercise we perform optimises or hinders our movement. We can make people move better or worse through specific instructions. If the human gait cycle (walking) of each individual is not accounted for, we can give them a potentially great programme, but one unsuitedto them that will inevitably lead to injury, stiff joints, fatigue and a poor quality of life.

I am not trying to scare you with this statement, but rather open your eyes to the possibilities when you have appropriate and structured exercise regimes. We can change movement for better or worse, so use it wisely!

We have covered breathing, now let's talk motion!

A simple way to understand motion is to break it down into the components that we, as humans, have access to.

MOTIONS OF MOVEMENT

We have three basic motions of movement that we call planes. The sagittal, frontal and transverse. Inside these three planes exists the entirety of human movement. These planes split movement up into easily understandable patterns. If you utilise planes of motion within your programming, you can create effective, fun and results-based exercises to enhance your capacity to move well.

Similarly, if we only focus on one plane for too long i.e., a powerlifting style that revolves around one plane (sagittal), we can inhibit movement. Now, this isn't to say a powerlifting style is bad.

Powerlifting-style training consists of three primary movements: bench press, squatting and deadlifting. The theme that underlies these movements is requiring the use of both of either your arms or legs. When you squat, you bend both legs, then extend both legs to get you upright again.

If this is all you do when training, without respecting other patterns, what can you foresee happening? Often, we find that powerlifters become extremely adept at these skills and the sagittal plane but lose their athleticism; their ability to change direction, walk, run, jump.

To the powerlifters out there, as we will discuss within the movement programming section, your accessory movements may make or break your programme. If you want to still be capable of moving extreme weights but also walk down the street or up a flight of stairs, put some weight in your accessories!

This will still enable people to get the best of both worlds. Other sports may dictate a bias towards certain planes as well, and this is ok within the context of sport. This will, in fact, be required to achieve an elite level within the constrained demands of that sport. For the general population, however, people who just want to move and feel better need balance across all three planes.

So, what are these planes and what movements exist in each?

Sagittal Plane

Imagine cutting someone into two equal halves lengthways – left and right (anterior (front) and posterior (back)); think of any movements that cause you to flex and extend or, in other words, bend and straighten.

These movements might be deadlifts, jumping, walking, bicep curls. This is the most common plane of movement that is programmed. As mentioned above, a powerlifting programme will generally focus on the sagittal plane.

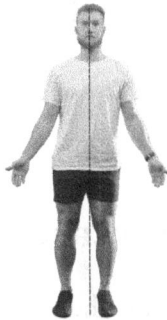

Sagittal

Figure 2.1

Frontal Plane

Can you guess this one? Frontal plane refers to the front; in fact, it splits the body into front and back halves and involves motion in and out (adduction and abduction). Exercise examples may Include lateral raises, crab walks, bending to the side.

This is often an important plane to assess someone's gait when walking and running. Here we can see how the body rotates,

spins and drops through compensation or what the person ac-
cesses to accomplish the task in front of them.

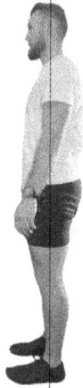

Frontal

Figure 2.2

TRANSVERSE PLANE

The last plane of motion – the transverse – is an interesting
one that I often see neglected in the majority of programming.
This is, nonetheless, still a crucial plane which works through
horizontal rotation. If we took your body and cut it in half
across the middle, we get the transverse plane (superior (top) and
inferior (bottom)).

This one took me a while to wrap my head around, so I will try
and break it down in a simple, easy-to-understand way.

Imagine a sport that involves both halves of the body. For me,
I like to visualise cricket or golf. Both of these sports involve
rotation. We cross our body in both of these sports by rotation
through our feet, hips (inferior) and thoracic spine (superior).
Motions within this plane, if we are thinking of the gym, include:

wood chops, thoracic rotation mobility and pronation/supination exercises of the forearm and feet.

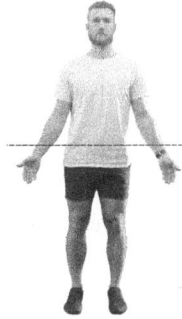

Transverse

Figure 2.3

WHAT ARE THE BENEFITS OF BEING MINDFUL OF THE PLANES OF MOTION?

Well, first let's think back to everyday movement – for this example, we will imagine you decide to make the most of a beautiful summer day and hang out some washing to dry (fun, right?).

You walk forward (sagittal plane) towards your clothesline and the washing basket on the floor. You stand next to the washing basket and bend down and sideways (frontal) to grab some clothes. You hear someone call your name from behind, so you rotate your head and upper back to look behind you (transverse).

In this simple example, we have used all the planes of motion during an everyday task. We carry out thousands of these every day, whether that's reaching across our desk, picking objects up from the floor or checking our blind spots when driving. If we want to create an effective programme, one that allows us to move into and out of each of these planes when required, we need to incorporate all three planes of motion.

Incorporating this 3D model of movement into our exercise regime isn't just a means of preventing injury, rather it's a way to fulfil your potential! Through intelligent programming, we are enabling our bodies to claim, or in some cases reclaim, patterns to achieve our goal, whether that's cycling the Tour de France or household chores like mowing the lawn. If we become fixated around one plane, as we demonstrated with the sagittal example, we restrict motion to the confines of that plane. We can get away with this for a while, but not if we want longevity for our joints and musculature.

WALKING GAIT

Walking, again, like breathing, is a pattern so many of us take for granted and butcher. However, I must admit this is also a testament to the adaptability of the human body: being able to overcome whatever life throws at you, and still being able to move, is impressive.

The normalcy or the notion of normalcy when it comes to the human gait cycle exists due to how our bone structure and muscles act. We are obviously not efficient and effective at walking on all fours; we have two legs that allow us to ambulate our environments in a more succinct manner.

If we are to break down the human gait cycle of walking into specific sub-components, – we find that two stages can explain majority of the walk –the stance and swing phases, as shown in Figure 2.4.

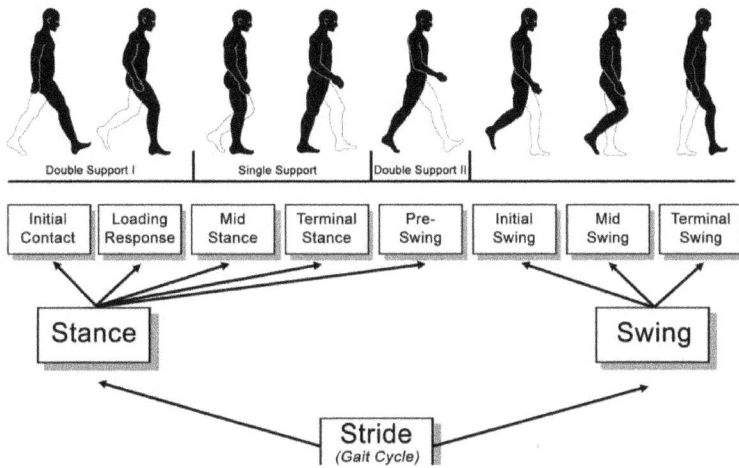

Figure 2.4

STANCE PHASE

The stance phase makes up the majority of forward motion, accounting for roughly 60% of the gait cycle. The stance phase can be broken down into a further three categories: initial contact, midstance and late stance.

Let's look at this from the bottom, working our way upwards. For this example, let's use just the right leg, as shown in Figure 2.4

During 'initial contact' – Phase 1 – we aim to strike the floor with our right heel, meaning our toes are up facing towards the roof, our pelvis is externally orientated and the opposite arm (left) will swing forward to counterbalance us. If we go back to our inhalation strategy, what does this sound like?

That's right – initial contact can be viewed as expansion: our foot is supinated and plantar flexed, our hip is abducted and externally rotated and flexed.

As we move through from the initial contact into the 'mid stance' – Phase 2 – our right foot eccentrically controls our weight down towards the floor, our pelvis internally rotates, our opposing arm falls by our side and we begin to shift our centre of gravity over the right foot. This occurs while the opposing leg transitions into the swing phase. This now references the compression stage as our foot pronates, our pelvis internally rotates around the standing leg's thigh bone (femur) and we extend our hip to centre us.

The third and final phase within the stance component of walking is to propel us forward, better known as the 'late' stance. Now that the weight is centred over our right foot, our foot is flat, and our knee and hip is extended (midstance).

To propel us forward we must re-plantarflex (raise our calf) with our right foot, our right hip goes back into external rotation and hyperextension and our opposing arm shifts behind our body. These processes enable us to move forward from late stance and into the next part of gait, where the whole process repeats itself with the left leg instead.

Basically, a simplified version is to think of walking as starting out (initial contact), going in (mid stance) and going back out (late stance).

SWING PHASE

This is when our leg is up in the air. Within the swing phase, our leg (let's make it the left one this time) acts a pendulum. This part of our gait does not take much energy (roughly 10-15% of the total energy expenditure required to walk).[3]

The left lower leg will move through four cycles:

- Pre-swing (transition between stance and swing).

- Initial swing (where our hip, knee and ankle are flexed to allow our foot to clear the floor).

- Mid-swing (when our thigh transitions forward).

- Terminal swing (when we begin extending our leg in preparation for initial contact to begin the next gait cycle).

The stance and swing phases combine to create a stride. That is one complete revolution of a leg from each time it lands.

Within our normal walking pattern above, an array of problems can occur. To list them all would require an encyclopedia longer than this book, so instead I will simply name a few of the big hurdles that impact our gait that I've experienced during my time as an exercise physiologist.

INJURY

We adopt what is referred to as an antalgic gait to prevent us from feeling pain in an injured area. Antalgic gait can be thought of as a way of moving that doesn't cause you as much pain as previously.

Think about a lower limb injury you may have had, an ankle sprain or knee pain such as patellar tendonitis maybe?

You will have changed how you walked to avoid the pain caused by placing weight on this injured body part. Now, acutely this is fine, but when this is left unchecked and becomes chronic, we may have an issue. We start to disproportionately strain other joints and segments and create what is one of the most overused words in the health and fitness world: 'overload'.

However, we can use this to our advantage. People that suffer from ankle, knee and hip pain can learn or relearn gait mechanics and prevent overloading of their joints. This is a suitable approach for those with conditions such as osteoarthritis and those afflicted with neurological conditions such as multiple sclerosis.[4]

BIOMECHANICS

Learning to walk is beautiful. It is a process during which we fall repeatedly, pick ourselves back up and learn the fine line between balance and mobility. Our body has developed and taken shape to allow our legs to swing, stand and everything in between. This doesn't always occur; people may be born with larger hip widths (e.g., females) resulting in a changed Q-angle (femur angle). Typically, due to having this from birth, our body will organise itself in a way that becomes accustomed to the biomechanics. Is it as efficient as the ideal gait we spoke about? Probably not, but it's enough to get the job done. Again, our bodies are highly adaptable, so we can adopt antalgic gaits to allow us to continue moving – it might not always be the ideal solution to the problem though.

GENETICS/ ILLNESS

As I alluded to moments ago, people that are afflicted with neurological conditions such as cerebral palsy, multiple sclerosis, Parkinson's disease, dementia or strokes can have altered gait patterns. While these conditions can be extremely debilitating and affect a cascade of mechanisms within the human body, their gait can still be improved through a combination of neuromuscular training, balance and global strengthening of their bodies. They may not achieve an aesthetically perfect gait cycle, but they can definitely achieve a more functional state leading to less stiffness, pain and compensation.

AGE

As we age, our bodies change. Lean body mass declines due to the atrophy of muscle cells.[5] Strength declines and balance and coordination become impaired. This can result in an altered gait; one I frequently see elderly people adopt is shuffling. The 'late' part of the stance phase where propulsion occurs is underused, and instead they shuffle to decrease the distance their feet need to move. This, in turn, most likely contributes to their heightened risk of falling – because their toes aren't clearing the floor, as per a normal gait during the initial contact of the foot (refer back to the image). Now they land with their toes on the floor, increasing the probability of stubbing their toe, leading to a tumble, trip or fall.

ASSESSING GAIT

Each of the factors listed above are important not just for gait changes but knowing how to programme specific exercises to enable improved quality of movement. When assessing a walking pattern, I recommend that you **film the subject**. At fast speeds, the human eye can and will miss erroneous movements, no matter how good you are. Filming a subject, even with just a phone (most have decent enough cameras these days), will allow you to break down their gait so you can see exactly what is going on and in which phase of the gait this is occurring. You can break it down and watch it 100 times until you notice issues, if you're that way inclined.

At the time of writing this I frequently use an app – *Coach's Eye* – that enables me to slow down, draw on and compare multiple angles of walking time synced at once! There are plenty of programmes out there, but at the end of the day, your normal camera will be enough for the task at end.

Now, when filming how you walk, here are some recommendations:

- Make sure you capture enough of yourself moving, at least a couple of strides. Setting up the camera about 6-7 metres away from where you will start walking is sufficient to get what you need.

- Make sure you film multiple angles e.g., if looking at the sagittal plane, walk within the constraints of the camera both right and left. If looking at the frontal plane, then walk towards the camera and then away from the camera. Frontal and sagittal planes will show different errors in the gait. Make sure to capture both planes as you will miss movements when only viewing in 2D.

- Ensure you have good lighting! Is it too dark, too bright or too glary? Are you wearing black clothing? Good luck seeing anything. Make sure you have the right conditions to film clear and crisp video footage.

- Take time to analyse the video, especially if you are new to breaking down movement. If you rush it or jump to conclusions, you will miss things. These can be small or big issues, and if you focus on the wrong segment, you may not get the desired outcome.

FRONTAL PLANE

This is vital for assessing how well people rotate during the gait cycle. Throughout this position we can view the ankles to look at how well they pronate and supinate, how the pelvis internally and externally rotates and what happens with this person's trunk as they move through the gait cycle.

Sagittal Plane

This is our forward and backward motion, best seen by watching the individual move from their side. Set the camera up again, 20 feet away from the subject, and film them walking from side on. This will allow you to establish whether the ankles, knees, hips and arms move through extension and flexion.

Running Gait

We've covered the walking gait, the stance and swing phases that propel us forward, the way heel striking occurs at initial contact followed by plantarflexion (calf raise) of the foot during the late stance phase to move us into the second half of our stride. Walking will always occur with at least one foot in contact with the ground at all times.

Running has different parameters. Running is often defined as having a period of no ground contact, or 'flight'.[6] This flight refers to both limbs being off the floor, followed by ground initial contact. With this initial contact there can be significant differences: people can land with the heel, mid-foot or forefoot once initial contact has occurred.

It's my belief that mid-foot to forefoot running is preferrable to a heel-strike pattern. Research on this subject is limited and inconclusive at the time of writing, with neither forefoot- or heel-striking proving superior for energy economy or injury prevention.[7,8] In my experience, which is backed by research, injuries such as shin splints, iliotibial band pain, patellar tendinopathies and Achilles tendinopathies can be treated through altering the gait parameters of an individual.[9,10]

Now, this isn't to say forefoot running will solve your issues instantly and prevent all pain. Remember that the forefoot is the first point of contact of your distal limb, and there are still a host of issues that can occur, such as a weak or immobile forefoot, changes in the joint positions above the foot/ankle and compensations. The reason I will focus on forefoot strike is to encourage appropriate load transfer between the ankle, knee and hip and back as we transition through our strides. Landing with a heel strike encourages a flexed foot, with an extended knee and hip vs. a forefoot strike which encourages a partially flexed knee and hip joint. I will often give the example of jumping. If you stand up and jump up and down on the spot, think about how this feel.

I can wait.

Ok, you're back?

Now, try jumping again, only this time absorb the force by allowing a soft bend in your knee and hip, almost as if you are starting to lower onto a chair.

Feel the difference?

With the latter scenario, we have changed our joint kinematics, increasing the movement of our arms, joint angles and the surface area of force absorption.[11,12] By allowing our joints to bend, as opposed to adopting a stiffer, extended position, we can mitigate the force on our joints. Running can transfer a load of four or five times your body weight onto your joints.[8] We need to spread this load out, and that is exactly what I aim to do when re-educating runners around their gait mechanics.

Running is an art. Beautiful if done correctly, a disaster if done poorly. Running for many is used as an effective cardiovascular workout, a recreational and competitive activity. Running to me is an illustration of the body's ability to coordinate, control and display force across multiple joints in a timely manner to formulate a pattern. An area we will discuss in detail is isometrics, how these are used and where we can find them in everyday movements such as running.

Putting this all together we can view human locomotion as the accumulation of body segments, working in unison to achieve motion.

If you're looking to begin running, another important consideration is the speed at which you run. This is known as cadence or how many times your foot touches the floor per minute. A good cadence is between approximately 170-190 beats per minute (bpm). This will reduce your ground contact time, increase your springiness and decrease your injury risk.

Cadence Coach is an app I use to manually track how many steps someone I'm assessing is taking. Another rule of thumb is that change takes time. Don't aim too high or you will end up like Icarus and crash. Instead, have patience and build your running cadence slowly. Try to increase by roughly 10% of your total per week.

For example, if your cadence is 130 bpm, add 13 bpm the next week and so on until you find a comfortable pace that you can maintain.

3

Preparation Is Success

Give me six hours to chop down a tree and I will spend the first four sharpening the axe." -Abraham Lincoln

Have you ever tried to exercise without a decent warm-up? Chances are you might find your joints feeling stiff, achy even, maybe you feel sluggish at the beginning of your exercise or maybe you just go through the motions at the beginning of the session. This is why I've dedicated this chapter to the pre-movement variables that should be taken into account.

How we prepare for movement dictates how our session will go. This holds true not just in the gym, but for all exercises, sports and activities in life. We need a certain level of preparedness to be able to engage and perform at an adequate or optimal level.

This involves identifying a few key variables that we must account for if we wish to achieve our best output for the chosen activity: the movements or skills involved, how our body is feeling, our weaknesses and strengths, time constraints and our mindset.

Getting the most out of your activity starts with the warm-up!

The warm-up is designed to, you've guessed it, warm us up! At least, this is what it should be doing. Physiologically speaking, it involves stimulating blood flow to the relevant area.

This occurs by increasing our heart rate, blood pressure and stroke volume, which is key to increasing our heart's working capacity. Have you ever felt your heart racing? Maybe you sprinted for a short amount of time, ran up a flight of stairs or you were anxious about an upcoming event?

In these cases, our bodily systems – the cardiovascular, musculoskeletal, respiratory, nervous and metabolic –work together to allow us to adapt to our environment. The cardiovascular system, that is our heart, veins and arteries, changes how it operates to allow more or less oxygen to reach our muscles to match our required activity. Processes such as vasoconstriction and vasodilation, which are essentially expansion and compression, occur within the veins and arteries to regulate how much blood we can move through our body.

We may start breathing faster (ventilation rate increases) and take in more oxygen (ventilation volume increases) through our respiratory system, which allows for greater gas exchanges between the blood and lungs to encourage more oxygen to be supplied to our musculoskeletal system and cardiovascular system.[13]

Our muscles are now being supplied with more blood and oxygen, which will increase their temperature and reduce stiffness, allowing our musculoskeletal system to exert more force.[14,15]

Our nervous system works through energy to stimulate our muscles. We can be excited (high energy current) or fatigued (low energy current). With a warm-up, our nervous system will become 'primed' toward a high-energy current. Think of priming as starting your car and letting the engine go idle, it's ready for action. Priming relies on the sympathetic pathway to exhibit fight or flight within the autonomic nervous system. A response may be to breathe faster, taking in more oxygen for the muscles to work when required. This increases our ability to produce force and create the optimum environment for muscle contractions.[16]

Our metabolic system will alter the number of hormones we produce and secrete to supply energy to our bodily systems to sustain the output; glucagon, a form of carbohydrate, will be released to richly supply our blood with energy for exercise.[17,18]

Having all our systems primed and ready to face the demands of our sport or activity will even reduce our risk of injury.[19] If you are still debating whether you should warm up, please re-read the above section and let it sink in. The benefits are clear, and these are just some of the physiological mechanisms that will occur unconsciously during a well-executed warm-up

The key term I used just then was 'well-executed'. The physiological effects described may not occur, or at least to the capacity they should. If we don't warm up with solid intent, structure or thought behind how or why are doing it in the first place. Going through the motions and just moving for the sake of moving is not effective. I call this performing mindless repetitions. We must be aware of what we are doing and be mindful of how we are moving our body, making it a conscious process. This is certainly true for stretching, which I will cover later.

Have you ever walked into the gym, looked around at what's available and jumped on the nearest free piece of equipment? This might have been some form of cardiovascular machine: a treadmill, bike, elliptical or rower. You might have gone to the gym with the intention of improving your upper body strength and size. Instead of priming our musculature for an upper body workout, we simply walk on a treadmill and then immediately start our upper body movements.

Is this the best way to get ready for our session? Most likely not. Just like our training programmes, we must be selective with our warm-up activities. People will often start off with foam rolling, some basic static stretches and perform the same old movements a hundred times. Almost like a pattern, wouldn't you say? As humans, we are pattern-orientated, so it is easy to fall into the trap of what's familiar and rely on our habits because that's what we've always done.

What's missing here? Intent, direction and a little bit of novelty.

Our warm-up is intended to prime us for the activity. Through a burst of concentration and intensity, we can warm ourselves up physically and mentally, reduce our injury risk and prompt the physiological adaptions mentioned previously.

Direction refers to knowing what needs warming up to get the most out of our session. Rather than simply walking on a treadmill before an upper body session, we should look at what we are actually training e.g., selecting movements that mimic the chosen patterns, such as bench presses and bent-over rows. We should pay attention to what our body is telling us when coming into a session. Maybe our shoulders are feeling stiff. Start in this area, or at least straight after that walk on the treadmill if you still enjoy doing that. This will give you the ability to get that much-needed blood flow to the relevant area, supplying it with nutrients and fresh oxygen so you can be at your best. Think of this like micro-peaking for the event of your day.

Adding some novelty is doing something new, something fresh. We know that patterns are created through performing high repetitions and repeating tasks over and over until the neurons 'wire and fire together'. In essence, you are becoming autonomous or a master of this pattern. There is a catch, though: not all autonomy is good autonomy. In fact, if we perform the same warm-up routine over and over again, we switch off due to the anticipation of the patterns. This will lead to less intent and focus during the warm-up. Instead, look to change things up. Try a skill-based task, like juggling or rotating one arm forward and one arm back, then try more specific movements. Rather than just doing a few light sets of bench presses, try push-ups, triceps extensions and lat raises to warm the surrounding areas. Mix and match new movements every few weeks to give you variety, fun and, most importantly, an effective warm-up. There is no best warm-up for this very reason.

Have you ever performed a warm-up that feels just as long as the workout itself? Again, you are most likely not being effective here. If it takes too long to warm up, you may actually be cooling down by the time you get into the workout. As a rule of thumb, I will generally cap my warm-up movements at around three to four different ones or five to 10 minutes to ensure I do not burn up instead of warm-up. I do not waste needless energy on a warm-up that takes too long. Instead, I see it as a microdose of concentration to get me ready or in the zone for what's ahead of me.

MY WARM-UP PROCESS

I will keep my warm-ups simple yet directed, highly focused yet short.

I will aim to give myself some sensory form of movement, for example laying on my back and breathing, possibly elevating my legs so I can recalibrate my body for the upcoming movements. Think of this like a nap for the nervous system: rather than stressing after a day of work and trying to jump into the session, instead I will transition between nervous system states, tapping into the parasympathetic through some sensory breathing or grounding drills. Then I'll reengage with the sympathetic system.

I will then move into a pattern that may be foreign to me or that I suck at (the novelty). I will aim to explore my range of hip or shoulder motion, again through some form of ground-based movement. Much like brushing your teeth with your opposite hand, this will cause me to think, concentrate and become present with what I am doing so I can complete the task. This has both a psychological and physical priming effect on our bodies. Lastly, I will incorporate a movement that raises my core temperature and initiates the physiological processes we spoke about above. This may involve a large multi-joint movement or movements in succession to simulate activities that will be in my programme, something like jump squats or inch worms. Then I am ready for my workout. Short and sweet!

WHAT HEATS UP MUST COOL DOWN

If warm-ups enhance our physiological system to create greater output from basically all our bodily systems, the cooldown is the natural flow, the calming of our systems back to an energy-efficient state where we can get on with our low-level, everyday activities. Being amped or primed for too long can wreak havoc on our bodies. Chronic stress is an example of this, where we are essentially fixed in a state of fight or flight and our body is working overtime, or in other words, just keeps warming up. It's part of the reason why I dedicate time to tapping into my parasympathetic system.

Will this happen every time you miss a cooldown? Most likely not, but, over time, if we do not allow ourselves to relax and go back to our neutral state, issues can arise. This is a fact of life. We can only take on so much stress, work, family commitments, bills and social gatherings, all of which add to our stress levels. If our plate becomes too full, things will have to give way — often the first things are our mental and physical health. Take the time to recover so you can manage what is on your plate!

One way to do this is through an adequate cooldown. This relates to our autonomic, or parasympathetic, nervous system, namely rest and digestion. We tap into this state to downregulate our bodily systems: our breathing slows, our muscles relax, our blood lactate levels decrease, and our venous and arterial systems dilate decreasing the pressure within the arterial and venous walls and allowing our bodies to essentially rest and recover.[20] Generally, this is again specific to the activity. We may perform static stretches, breathing drills and gentle dynamic actions to allow our bodies to gradually come back to a normal resting state following bouts of movement.

Both warm-ups and cool-downs are essential physical activity components. Neglect one for too long and you risk injuries, causing your sessions and therefore your progression to slow over time and you will not achieve your goals in an effective manner. Cooldowns may be viewed as the precursor to recovery. A sufficient recovery lets you to engage with a stimulus that allows you to change (overreaching) and then recover to perform better next time (supercompensation). Without initiating the recovery process via a cool down, we risk overtraining – remember that big bad area we want to avoid?

ASSESSMENTS: WHO, WHAT, WHERE, HOW AND WHY?

Creating a tailored programme stems from a quality assessment. You may have been asking how do I know what the appropriate exercises are, how do I choose specific and tailored movements to enable the correction of my movement and how do I even know if my movement is not as good as it should be?

Drum roll ... The assessment.

Each of you reading or listening to this book will have a personal medical history, wants, needs and goals. These are what we call subjective components. Once we have a clear subjective understanding of you, we must move into the objective testing area. That is, performing a number of assessments to determine what exactly you need, what you have and what we need to do to allow you to reach your desired outcome or goal.

In the clinical world, practitioners would refer to a number of special tests, that is a series of movements designed to allow us to determine with differing accuracies whether a particular diagnosis is positive or negative. Within the general population, trainers may look at how someone squats, stands and performs tasks related to their sport or goal to determine what is required.

You will have different objective criteria if you play soccer vs. netball. Although there are some similar characteristics – jumping, running, changing direction – the overall commitments will be different.

Don't fall into the trap of pattern recognition, that is thinking once you have seen one person with knee pain, you have seen all people with knee pain. This can lead to cookie-cutter programmes that move away from client-centred approaches and towards a generic service, much like surfing Google to find a generic gym programme.

I generally view someone from the bottom up, top down. This means I will start at the feet, the base of support for all other structures, which allows me to move up their chain of movement command and delve into the intricacies of what may be underworking or overworking i.e., what is compensating and, more importantly, why.

My suggestion for your own personal assessment is to be global. Do not simply refer to the sight of pain or stiffness if you have any, look deeper. Think about your environment, the frequent tasks you engage in, and what your sport or daily tasks require of you. Think of yourself as a whole rather than apart.

We are but the summation of multiple joints working in unison to achieve a common goal. Imagine we have a clock and one of the interlocking becomes jammed and fails to carry out its purpose. How long do we imagine the clock will continue to work unhindered before another gear breaks down? Even though I used a machine for this analogy, it should be clear we are not machines and do not operate in a simple binary state of one thing works, and the other doesn't. Rather, we are complex multi-celled organisms, and the cause for our inability to move may be from our thoughts, feelings, environment (both past and present), how we manage our stress levels and a host of other reasons. People are complex.

With all that being said, are you still wondering what we are looking at?

I would assess the person's ability to flex, extend, rotate, move in and move out of positions, and how well they can reciprocate symmetry between their limbs. If one person has 30 degrees of internal shoulder rotation on one side but 70 degrees on the opposing side, we know their rib cage, scapular mechanics and breathing are going to be affected. From here we can break out further into more specific tests to figure out which gear in their body isn't performing its role. This involves utilising both subjective and objective measures. You might determine from the subjective assessment that they are a baseballer and commonly throw using one side, leading to greater internal rotation. Questions then arise about how much we should really change before we affect their performance.

COMMON GLOBAL AND LOCAL OBJECTIVE ASSESSMENTS I CARRY OUT INCLUDE:

- Toe touch or multi-segmental flexion

- Reaching above head or multi-segmental extension

- Squatting and hinging

- Supine shoulder range of motion – flexion, external and internal rotation, abduction and adduction

- Pelvic and ribcage orientation (motion in multiple planes, compression and expansion)

- Hip flexion, both bent and straight leg variations

- Knee flexion and extension

- Foot pronation and supination

- Hip internal/external rotation

These tests will give you a global view of the body; the majority of human movements exist within the above assessments. When we understand the role of our musculoskeletal system, the underlying anatomy and functionality of the human body provides numerous ways to test our capabilities.

If you were to present to me with knee pain, I will still look above and below, viewing both the hip and ankle. If someone presents with back pain, I will look above and below, assessing their hip mobility and control as well as the superior structures and how they are able to breathe and coordinate their ribcage with their pelvis. Those who view the body locally rarely treat the condition and, more importantly, prevent it from coming back or creating a new compensation altogether.

Now, this is a simple assessment. Once I have an understanding of the way someone can move their body, especially under my instruction, I start assessing their functional capacity. This involves strengthening and endurance-based measures, ideally throughout their entire body. For the general population, this involves observing their large movements in time-based and weight-based activities.

Due to my background and bias, I rely on variants of the big six patterns we spoke about earlier during my assessment of functional capacity. This may look like performing as many repetitions as possible within 30 seconds, for example, squats or push-ups. I will assess strength through unilateral means as well, that is give the subject dumbbells or kettlebells while they row or lunge to monitor potential imbalances within their body.

I expect asymmetry, which is inherent to the human body based on our anatomy. I'm not after perfect mirroring, although that would be nice. Instead, I utilise the limb symmetry index, especially with tasks like returning to sport or work, to determine if the difference between the performance of limbs from one side to the other is within 10%.

This gives some leeway for movement discrepancies e.g., if I got 30 reps on my left arm (dominant), I should be able to get 27 on my right (non-dominant).

Now, I said we are all asymmetrical. You may be scratching your head at this point. Is everyone obsessed with symmetry? Well, yes, but let me give you a quick insight into the human body.

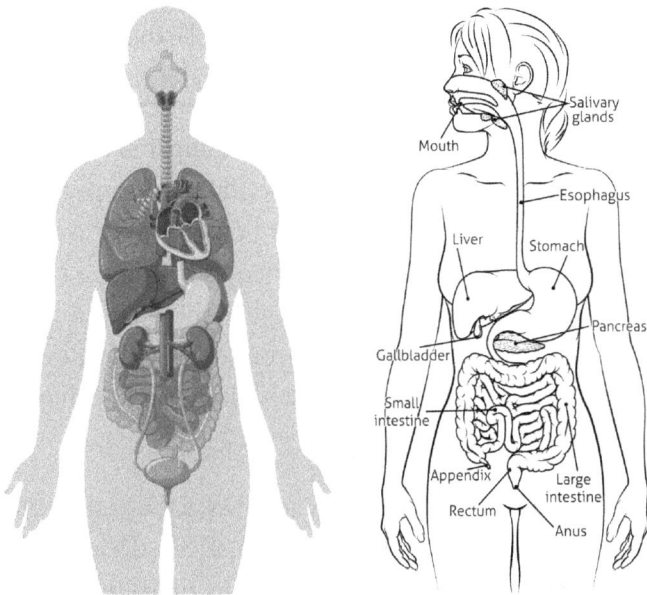

Figure 3.1

The image above (Figure 3.1) show the different layers of our bodies. We can see our right lung is larger compared to the left, having three lobes instead of two. This is to account for the heart being centred more to the left. The bulk of our liver is situated on the right side, where our colon, gallbladder and pancreas are also located. Knowing that the human body is inherently asymmetrical on the inside is important to understand, as it allows us to adapt different approaches for different parts of our body.

When performing tests, I am looking for symmetry in areas of strength and endurance of muscles, ideally this would present as the person completing the tests unilaterally within one or two repetitions for each limb, or 10%. For example, if I was testing using a DB chest press and the person's dominant side was the left, I would expect 10 reps on their left side and eight or nine reps with their right. Typical strength tests involve setting an arbitrary number of repetitions e.g., 10 reps and performing a maximum test to give us a baseline of their current capacity. Continue to increase the weight until 10 reps is unachievable, then note down the last successful attempt, which is their baseline capacity.

It's common to use 10 reps, which allows comparison with others, but if you need something more specific to your sport don't get hung up on that number. If you're a powerlifter, you will seldom need to perform 10 reps, so there isn't really a need to test it. I'd choose a much lower rep range in this instance to find out the relative baseline. For most of you reading this, however, 10 reps is an easy and safe range to test without too much risk of injury.

Strength tests will give me a few key insights, such as the psyche of the subject in relation to pushing themselves. Chances are if they are new to training, they will fall short of 10 reps. This is due to not having an anchor or a reference point for what they are capable of. It is very easy to stop when you feel the slightest discomfort.

Strength tests also show me what compensations the person may rely on during particular patterns, especially at certain points in time, and it allows me to gauge the appropriate relative intensities for the proceeding sessions for certain movements.

For clientele that require a more specific approach, such as athletes, I will aim to replicate the demands and constraints of their chosen sport to ensure my assessment is not only accurate but tailored to meet their specific needs. You can do the same by following the simple procedure below.

1. Know the sport – what is involved and for how long, the repeatability of the skill, and the planes of movement they work within (most sports will have most if not all).

2. What is the predominant energy system? Yes, each energy system will be active, but does their sport involve

lots of short bursts or continuous aerobic activity, for example?

3. What is the client's goal? (Where do they need to get to and how long do they have?)

4. Determine the tests based on information gathered in the first two steps to help them reach that goal.

5. Test using repeatable, realistic measures consisting of both subjective and objective metrics. Note their perceived exertion, skill quality, times, and rate of force development – whatever metrics you need. Then retest at appropriate intervals.

You will make mistakes, you will miss some data and you undoubtedly will misinterpret your findings (hopefully not all of these or it may be time to re-evaluate your process!). However, the fact that you will repeat the tests enhances your results because there is one consistent variable – you. This is often referred to as intra-rater reliability.

Nonetheless, making mistakes is a great way to learn! You should have a degree of self-reflection in every aspect in your life. Consistently aim to refine your testing measures so you get better at doing more with less. No assessment will fit every person, and that is ok. As long as you can get data that is meaningful to you, that in itself is better than not assessing at all. If you make a mistake and realise down the track, is it really the end of the world? In most cases, no. Strive for perfection, but expect mediocrity with your testing regime.

CHANGING THE BODY

There's a lot of negativity around corrective exercises, mostly, it seems to me, from people who have either not understood them or who have used the wrong ones. This is understandably frustrating, as people think they've done all this work to correct an area while unknowingly using the wrong approach.

The result is a negative association with the term correcting, so the next time you see a professional who says "Oh, you need to correct x, y and z", your mind will most likely think of your past experience and switch off.

So, what can we do? Is there even a corrective exercise out there?

A lot of the research will say no, with guidelines just encouraging movement in general. For the most part I agree, but I've always come across people who are scared of moving in the first place, so it never works to simply say you need to move more. This is where we must again look at the person as a whole using biopsychosocial and enactive approaches.

Let's explain what they are and how they differ.

BIOPSYCHOSOCIAL APPROACH

This is a popular model these days, one I have often used to establish how our body responds to stimuli. It basically consists of three concepts (biological, psychological and social) that allow us to identify reasons for issues in the body ranging from pain to behaviour and movement.

Biological refers to physical health, genetic predispositions and effects from external influences such as drugs. A simple way to think about this is someone born with a congenital condition such as spina bifida – the person has no influence, it is purely genetic or biological at this stage.

Psychological refers to concepts such as self-efficacy or self-esteem, e.g., how you are able to cope in different settings or environments. Think of this like learning how to cope with having spina bifida. You may have to complete tasks in a different way to the next person.

Social relates to how you interact with your peers, family and friends. Maybe you don't like going to parties due to the feeling that you won't fit in. This can lead to fear avoidance of certain activities.

Each of these three concepts can influence your body and movement as a whole. If we think we are incapable of a particular pattern or rely on other patterns due to a lack of efficacy, high anxiety or physical impairments, we become that person through wiring our neurons in that way.

ENACTIVE APPROACH

I consider this an updated biopsychosocial model, in that it explains how the above factors interact. It doesn't just follow a linear notion of causality, such as someone born with spina bifida struggles to cope in different environments, leading to social issues and the feeling of not belonging.

The enactive approach revolves around is the five Es:

- Embodied

- Embedded

- Enacted

- Emotive

- Extended

Each of these refer to how people interpret their current, past and future environments through the knowledge they gain in making sense of the world. It is a constant state of flux rather than the linear a + b = c. Each factor influences the other as we constantly grapple for understanding.

An example of this in practice could be someone with chronic back pain. This becomes the person's identity: they live, feel and breathe their back pain. Certain stimuli caused the onset of that pain. This pain is then regulated through the person's ability to make sense of this stimuli. This person will change their thoughts, behaviours and actions within their existing environment, for better or worse.

This model is still being fleshed out by researchers, so this will likely change moving forward. However, it does allow us to make sense of how these interactions can influence one another constantly on a theoretical level.

The point I want you to take away from the above concepts is to constantly take account of the body, mind and other factors like the environment when looking to change your movement. You will need to delve into your beliefs, how you spend the majority of your time, which of your nervous systems is predominant and so on. It is complex and takes time. Be patient and record what you think, feel and do across your day or week. This is the best approach to 'correcting your movement'.

A better term than correction is preparation, in my view. Preparation involves a specific exercise or combination of exercises to achieve the outcome of restoring your spectrum of movement.

You may ask the question, isn't all movement corrective in nature?

Well, no, not entirely. Early on I mentioned that exercise can be a powerful tool, to either enhance or decimate our bodies. Choosing the wrong exercises, or simply coaching the right exercises the wrong way, can reinforce poor patterning and create compensations in new areas of our bodies. This isn't life or death, but it can interrupt our progress and potentially place us at greater risk of injury if sustained for a decent period of time.

For me, the best way I can teach someone how to move is to have experienced that movement myself, so I can grasp what I should and shouldn't be feeling. Now, keep this within reason. No one will be perfect at every exercise, but at least view how the movement should be performed from multiple angles. Understand how you learn best, thinking back to the senses or visual, auditory, written or kinaesthetic learner archetypes. Establish your norms and have expectations around what is required when engaging in an exercise. Imagine explaining how to drive a car if you've only used a Hot Wheels set as a kid. You need to watch, experience and feel what it is like to actually drive a car to be able to explain it properly to someone else.

Preparation exercises by nature are generally slow and thoughtful. We are trying to stimulate strong neuronal connections to create a link to this pattern. If we rush through this, again we may compensate, hold our breath and miss the whole point of trying to breathe and live through new movements.

Through an accurate and thorough subjective assessment, we can avoid the above pitfalls and make lasting movement changes. Remember the power of the mind? If we have a negative outlook, why wouldn't the effects of the exercise be reduced – remember the nocebo effect? If it was poorly coached to us, if it wasn't actually the underlying cause of the compensation which led to our pain or stiffness, then of course it will not be effective from a biomechanical point of view.

Just as with assessments, preparation exercises should not be cookie-cutter. We should not say someone with back pain must do glute bridges; on what basis are we making this claim? While certain movements can definitely help, they must be used within the correct context. Maybe instead of glute bridges they need a bilateral approach or they need to focus on expanding a part of their ribcage, altering their bone and therefore allowing the length-tension relationships of the muscles to be restored. They may have reservations around movement i.e., fear avoidance, and unconsciously tense their body in anticipation, creating too much core tension. There are a thousand possible reasons, as we discovered through the biopsychosocial and enactive models. The contributing factors or underlying cause won't become apparent until we test.

We must assess to identify compensation patterns so we can diagnose and address any issue in an appropriate and selective way. We mustn't just suggest something because we have seen it work with another person before.

An example I frequently see is the assumption that people with back pain must have weak cores (most research suggests the opposite is true). These people deemed as having a weak core will be given exercises such as the supine 90/90 positions similar to that of a dead bug, which has become insanely popular throughout the fitness community. Now, research indicates that most of these people don't actually need increased core strengthening, so this exercise will be ineffective for them even though it's deemed 'corrective'. Sure, it might work for some people, but the point is that just because it is successful with one person, doesn't mean it will work for you and your individual needs. Always keep this in the back of your mind.

By now, hopefully, you will be aware that movement selection should not be taken lightly. If you are unsure of what is best for you, what will help you improve your quality of life and restore proper movement to your body, then find a quality coach that can properly assess what you need.

You should assess them as well! Ask questions, like:

What are their credentials?

Do they communicate in a way that you understand?

Do they tailor their exercises to you or give the same thing to all their clients?

I find people who often get the best results have one thing in common: they ask questions. They question the rationale of me providing them exercises. This allows them to understand why they are doing things rather than mindlessly performing reps. Understanding the why provides context, which translates into motivation and adherence. Adherence is king for being successful.

Hopefully, after reading this book, you will be on the path to becoming a better version of yourself and understanding the nuances of communicating, the thought behind selecting the right exercises and how to know when you aren't moving properly.

The main purpose of the preparation exercise is simply to give people what they do not possess. If someone is anteriorly pelvically tilted (this is where your sacrum or centre of your pelvis pushes forward), they will likely be capable of decent internal thigh rotation, but lack external rotation and decent heel contact.

If someone can expand their ribcage anteriorly (front) when breathing but lacks posterior expansion, they will need reaching-based movements to encourage posterior expansion to restore their normal spinal curvature e.g., thoracic kyphosis and cervical and lumbar lordosis. You get the drift. In my experience, people at the extremes get there by neglecting the opposing spectrum of movement. Remember our doorway analogy? We want to find the centre, to move in and out, left and right, up and down. If we are too far towards one end of our spectrum, it is very difficult to get to the other side.

LENGTH AND TENSION

The length-tension relationship states that each muscle within our body has an optimal position to produce force. It relies on the spectrum of stretching and shortening and finding the equilibrium between these two points. It has been made famous through pioneers such as Janda, a physiotherapist and founder of dynamic neuromuscular stabilisation, who proposed the upper and lower crossed syndromes. That is, if one muscle is tight, the antagonist muscle will be lengthened. Irrespective of how that holds up with research today, the fact remains that our muscles can produce force when they are positioned correctly.

We can use this length-tension relationship to impact movement. The classical model tells us to stretch a muscle for, say, 30 seconds for a repeated number of times, but I don't find this to be an effective way of stretching.

You may be thinking I'm crazy, but hear me out. Let's say I want to stretch my hip flexors because I am in an anterior pelvic tilt and my hips just feel tight overall. In line with the length-tension relationship, we know that the hip flexors will be shortened with an anterior pelvic tilt. So far, so good. Now, a common way to stretch this hip flexor is to drop down to one knee, basically in a lunge position, and push my hips into hip extension with the intent of putting the pelvis into a neutral position or even posterior pelvic tilt.

This process is known as reciprocal inhibition. We contract the muscle, causing it to shorten, and the opposing or antagonist muscle must do the opposite (lengthen) e.g., you tense your bicep in the front of your arm, causing it to shorten, and your triceps on the other side of your arm will stretch. By holding this hip-flexor stretching position for 30s, I will likely feel a nice stretch in my hip flexor before standing back up and carrying on with my day. By the end of the day my hips are tight again. The next day I repeat the same stretch, and I continue to do this over and over; my hips are forever tight, and I continue to stretch in that half-kneeling, hip-flexor position to give me some form of relief in my hips.

What's missing?

Why is it that I am unable to make meaningful and, more importantly, lasting change with this stretch? I've followed the lower-crossed syndrome approach and stretched what is tight. I may even implement some hip extension exercises because I feel my glutes are weak, and yet, at the end of all of this, I still have no change.

The missing components are the brain, the bones, our nervous system and our lifestyle. We have failed to address the underlying cause behind why the pelvis is tight. In the health and fitness industry, we are obsessed with tight muscles. All emphasis is placed on stretching muscles in a mindless way to try and create change within our body. Much like our warm-ups, we must have intent and direction when trying to change.

If our pelvis is orientated in an anterior pelvic tilt (front is lower than the back of the hips) in an upright position, how is our centre of mass displaced? Remember, the role of our body is to keep us upright: our body will twist, turn, bend and find the path of least resistance to do this. If we are in an anterior pelvic tilt, we must look at where our weight is shifting to cause this. A significant amount of people will be orientated over the front of their feet. They will lean forward over their toes, causing the hips to shift backwards and the torso to shift upwards to prevent them from falling over. This is called counterbalance. We will move one segment of our body in opposition to a segment above or below, essentially to allow us to stay balanced. It works for

a short period of time at the expense of altering our muscles'
length- tension relationship.

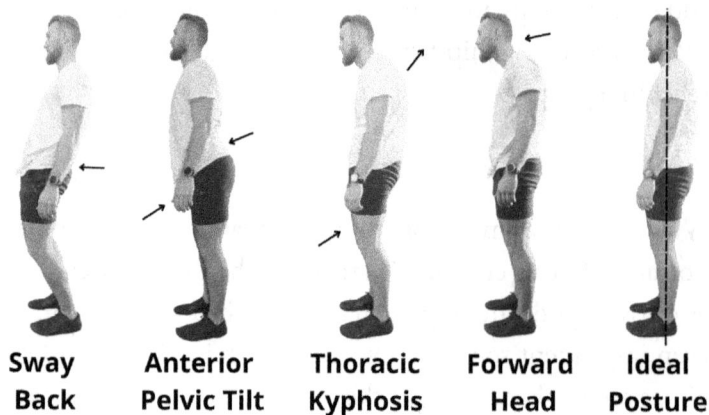

| Sway Back | Anterior Pelvic Tilt | Thoracic Kyphosis | Forward Head | Ideal Posture |

Figure 3.2

As you can see in Figure 3.2, a change in how we shift our weight
drastically changes our standing posture. Go to your nearest
shopping centre and start people-watching; you will notice the
body stands in a variety of different positions. This is a testament
to our innate ability as humans to adapt to and withstand the
pressures of gravity that are constantly trying to keep us down.

Our centre of gravity is a pivotal concept that must be fac-
tored in when aiming to improve movement. Instead of simply
stretching what is tight and strengthening what is weak, we must
integrate the nervous system, the brain and the bones to teach
ourselves the ideal 'centre' or neutral position for our muscles to
rest.

So, again, how do we achieve this?

Well, one of the ways is through neuromuscular training. That
is, placing ourselves into positions repeatedly while focusing our
attention on the intrinsic way our body organises itself. This

is how we change things on a cellular level and elicit neural adaptation within the brain.

An example of this may be to stand side on next to a mirror (ideally, a full-body mirror). Next, practice shifting your centre of mass through your feet. Think of Michael Jackson's anti-gravity lean forward as you place more weight over your toes; then, try the opposite, shifting back onto your heels. You will notice some subtle and not-so-subtle shifts in the surrounding joints of the knee, hip and shoulder to enable you to stay upright. You may even be a spitting image of some of the postures in Figure 3.2!

Learning how to spread weight evenly is the first step in becoming aware of how to change your posture. Doing this with your static posture isn't even close to enough when altering your body position long term, however, so don't expect amazing results from this simple exercise.

Neuromuscular training is a viable way to encourage you to live with your new movement capabilities. It differs from strength training largely through the act of being conscious and concerned with intrinsic mechanics.[21] It should involve placing the subject in positions similar to those they can't achieve and encouraging them to be consciously aware of how their body is responding to this. This will promote the quality and efficiency of movement.

One example of how this might look could be to lay on your back, place your heels on a step and lift your bum off the floor. Think of tucking your pelvis under, like you're trying to scoop an imaginary belt buckle up from the floor. This is great for giving people a sense of shifting weight onto their heels. An exercise like this gives you a sense of how the body would react to standing with heel contact (the first part of gait) but in a less aggressive way, as you are working perpendicular to gravity rather than against it. From here, you can try more complex tasks, like moving your arms, pumping your feet back and forth or marching to alternate your legs on the step.

Another useful technique is proprioceptive neuromuscular facilitation, or PNF training if you don't want to say that mouthful. This involves making your stretches active instead of passive. In this instance, we define active stretches as ones where you are conscious and creating force to make a change, rather than a passive approach of having no intent behind it.

To make sense of this concept, let's look at the following scenario.

To actively stretch your quads, lie face down and tie a band or towel around your foot. Then, wrap it over your shoulder and pull your heel towards your bum. While you're doing this, I want you to create resistance by trying to straighten your leg at the same times as your arms bend. This creates force, or active tension. Perform the holds for 5 to 10 seconds before relaxing moving further into the stretch and repeating the same active resistance.

A passive approach for stretching your quadriceps would be to simply pull your heel towards your bum and hold it there for 30 seconds without any active resistance. While this can be a valuable technique, we should ultimately move away from just stretching muscles in static positions and place more emphasis on the bones, respiratory and neuromuscular systems. A useful phrase for remembering how to make changes to your body is: **"The joints act and the muscles react."**

This means if you anteriorly tilt your pelvis, the surrounding musculature like the hip flexors, hamstrings, gluteal and adductors will shorten or lengthen in reaction to the change in bone orientation, and vice versa. If we move into a posterior or scooped-bum orientation, our body will instinctively alter the muscle tension again to allow us to sustain that position. In our above stretching example, we haven't worried about our pelvic orientation, only the muscles. So, when we stand up from our stretch, our quads will react to whatever orientation is present and either shorten or lengthen as a result. Always consider the bone and the desired outcomes. To make the above stretch better, I would encourage the bum to be tilted or pushed down into the floor as you bend your heel towards your bum to encourage the ideal bone orientation for the stretch.

An ideal standing position, as mentioned previously, is being stacked. This refers to having our centre of mass over our ankle bones (malleolus), our knee joint (epicondyles) situated over the ankle, with the pelvis, the shoulder and ears also in alignment as we transition higher up the body. This is ideal to put our muscles in the optimal resting length-tension positions, but will shift depending on the context. Once you have found the so-called ideal standing position, then you can make those muscles of yours shorten or lengthen as you desire.

To create our desired outcome in muscle tension, the key point I want you to remember is to make it an active process. Tap into your conscious mind and control your body rather than simply trying passive approaches like massage and static stretches. Don't get me wrong, I'm not bashing passive therapies like physiotherapy or osteopathy, they have a place and need. However, when it comes to enhancing the quality of your movement, active approaches will be more effective.

Our breathing is again important here. This must match our movement. If we are in a state of sympathetic activation when trying to stand in our new positions, our breathing with become rapid or possibly even stop. This is not beneficial for stimulating change. Call up the parasympathetic nervous system through controlled breathing so you can relax into these positions. This, in essence, is a message to your body and unconscious that you can live and survive in these muscle positions.

The result? Lasting postural change, allowing our muscles and bones to move freely within their full range of motion. We must tap into the pathways that create lasting postural change so we do not have to waste time performing the same stretches over and over, which at best give us positional rather than global change.

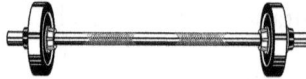

TIME TO RECAP!

- Warm-ups are essential for priming our physiology so we can perform at our peak.

- Cool-downs are essential for aiding our recovery and tapping into our parasympathetic nervous system.

- Assessments should be specific to you. Focus on subjective and objective measures to get a broad view of your history.

- Our body is asymmetrical – aim for similarity (within 10% of each limb), not perfection.

- To make LASTING change in the body, we must make global changes that account for the biological, psychological, social aspects, as well as how we make sense of our past, present and future experiences.

- Our body is constantly adjusting, keeping us upright by altering the length and tension of muscles in response to how we orient our bone structures.

- Choose active strategies like neuromuscular exercises

rather than passive massage therapies to create lasting movement enhancements.

- The breath must be incorporated into any attempt to alter the body. Other strategies involve neuromuscular training, which encourages conscious thought of how your body is reacting.

4

Stability Vs. Mobility (Ding Ding)

"Human movement is an amazing orchestra of muscle contractions controlled by the central nervous system to create joint actions to accomplish specific tasks"
-Mary Miller

S tability and mobility, is a concept I first discovered thanks to Gray Cook, one of the founders of the functional movement screen (FMS). This introduced me to the notion that our joints have specific roles, a chain of command, a segmental ebb and flow to encourage proper biomechanical motion. The spectrum of stability and mobility can be seen through the demands of sports and everyday life activities. Take an elite gymnast, who can perform amazing feats with how they move their body: they will have exceptional mobility and stability to perform within the constraints of their sport. Now, compare that to your average office worker, a person who lacks the mobility to be able to even touch their toes.

The principles of stability and mobility can be simplified by looking at our joints. The first joint should be quite rigid, strong and stable (stability joint). Both the proceeding and preceding joint above and below should be the opposite: malleable, unstable and free (mobility joint). Ideally, joints are organised in this alternating fashion between the spectrum of stability and mobility to create our functioning bodies and enabling the gift of motion.[22]

A joint is two bones that connect with one another. Starting from your ankle, I want you to try and draw a circle with your foot. To do this we need high degrees of mobility at the ankle (mobile joint). Now, try and do this with your knee joint – you can't. While it can move, it is not as mobile as the ankle joint. The knee joint instead is a rigid powerhouse (stable joint). Let's keep moving up the body and draw circles with our hip. This should be comfortable, and we should be able to create large circles because our hip is a mobile joint. Next, let's go to your lumbar spine or lower back. We have limited mobility again, but a nice broad stack of vertebrae to absorb load from (stable joints). Moving towards the upper thoracic spine we gain motion (mobility). I think you get the point.

If one joint is stable, the next will be mobile.

Are you following?

This is a concept that can be applied to an array of different injuries, movement deficiencies and patterns that allow us to move. When using this model to explain an injury, overload, strain, or whatever you wish to call it, there is often a breakdown in the above segmental chain of command. Take the knee, for example: an anchor between two mobile joints (the ankle and hip).

Now, after I sprained my ankle and it became as stiff as a rock, I have a goal of walking from one side of my house to the other. How am I going to do this?

My body says, "That's easy, I'll just start using other body segments and rely on them for the added motion required: We know from our breakdown of gait that we need varying degrees of ankle, knee and hip flexion and extension. If our ankle is stiff and we lose access to a range of flexion and extension (dorsiflexion and plantarflexion), we will fall over or injure our foot due to it scraping along the floor – unless we change. This is where our bodies shine; they are resilient and we subconsciously compensate to achieve our goals by adopting an antalgic gait.

This antalgic gait may present itself in the form of increased knee flexion during initial contact to account for the lack of dorsiflexion at the ankle during the gait cycle. This is an ideal scenario as we are giving the ankle a chance to recover through a reduced loading environment. Acutely, we need this. We need the body to recover promptly so we can return to our normal gait cycle.

Now, before I move on, let me put a question to you. Have you ever had an injury and said to yourself that you will just wait and do nothing until it heals? Maybe you actually saw a healthcare practitioner but didn't follow through with your rehab? Having learned earlier about the injury mechanisms that create our gait, can you now see why the reasons above can contribute to an abnormal cycle? Rehabilitation of the injured site is essential to prevent recurring or new injuries. Without following a decent rehabilitation protocol aimed at human locomotion, we place ourselves at a greater disposition towards compensation. Compensation, in my experience, cannot be maintained for long.

Antalgic gait is like having a friend over to your house; it's great to catch up and have them around, but as the day goes on and they don't leave they become more of a hindrance. Once our injury, in this case our ankle, has healed we should be loading it adequately with appropriate ranges of motion throughout the entirety of the gait cycle. When this ceases to occur, our once useful antalgic gait becomes our new full-time gait. Now, with the knee fulfilling an additional role of providing more mobility during the gait cycle, and the ankle acting as a stability point, we create a host of potential overloads, strains, additional compensations and so on until we get to a point where the pain becomes too much and we go and see someone about it.

This next paragraph is targeted at the practitioners of health care. This includes but is not limited to physiotherapist, chiropractors, osteopaths, kinesiologists, personal trainers and anyone else that is involved with human movement.

Adopt a holistic approach to your treatment. If we, as practitioners, choose to focus only on the site of injury we can miss the big picture, we can fail to rehabilitate people and we can lead them down the path of chronic injuries. I implore you to be a better practitioner, challenge your understanding and continually improve upon your knowledge of anatomy and physiology. Treatment that is outdated focuses purely on the local site of injury. We should now be practising global approaches to the enhancement and correction of human movement. We can apply models such as stability vs. mobility to understand the role of our joints in the body, for example if we see a really stiff hip and someone that has a tendonitis or another knee injury. Put two and two together and restore the proper segmental ebb and flow that we previously discussed. A broken chain will lead to greater issues the more distal we become from the location of injury. Have you just treated the site of the injury? You will get some results, but this will be short-lived. A quality subjective and objective assessment is required to gain as much information as possible regarding their medical history, injury timeline and approaches to healing so we can understand and truly treat their condition. Educate them about the injury, avoid scary jargon with your patients and desensitise them to their injury in a way that empowers them to take ownership of their health. Watch your patients flourish from here on out!

The physiological effects of having an unbalanced or inefficient joint disposition can lead to fatigue – we expend more energy to complete a task such as walking if we have an antalgic gait. We can experience increases in stress through the loading or overloading that occurs on joints acting out of character. This stress can lead to inflammation throughout the body, leading to conditions such as obesity, gout, gastrointestinal problems and heart disease.[23,24,25] We can cause chronic pain and stiffness when areas adopt new functions, presenting as anxiety, chronic fatigue, fibromyalgia and headaches to name a few.

Ok, you now know about stability and mobility and why it's important. Do you know how to use this information or test how a person's joints are working in their correct segmental path?

Stability and mobility go hand in hand; have you ever considered how they may affect each other? Stability, or a lack thereof, can greatly impede a person's mobility. Taking words straight from Gray Cook and Mike Boyle, "**we will sacrifice our mobility for stability**".

Refer to our three basic goals in life in Chapter 2. We want to first be able to breathe, next we want to stay upright and lastly move forward. To accomplish staying upright, we need stability. Stability is our anchor, it enables us to stand on one leg, climb stairs and walk on tight ropes (ok, maybe this last one isn't for everyone). Without stability we fall over. It is therefore in our bodies' best interest to do whatever is required to keep us stable; we will compensate, stiffen and contract areas of our body to do so. Let's take our unathletic office worker who is unable to touch their toes – is this a stability or mobility issue?

We can test this by giving them stability, an anchor point to hold onto or push off from, and then retest the pattern. If you put someone who cannot touch their toes into an upright position, then you place them in a sitting position ('long sit') and they can now touch their toes, that's a sure sign of a stability motor control dysfunction. Bit of a mouthful I know. Basically, this means that they are unable to adequately stabilise through their thoracolumbar (TL) junction, if we follow the joint-by-joint model mentioned earlier. In other words, when they reach for their toes, they feel unstable so their body reacts and tenses, and this tension limits their range.

If we gave them an object like a ball or pillow and placed it between their legs while they stood in an upright position, squeezing this object would provide them with stability through activating their intrinsic core musculature and surrounding tissues like their adductors. Now when they reach for their toes, almost like a magic trick, they will have increased their range and will instantly achieve a task they haven't in years or quite possibly their entire life.

If another person could not touch their toes in an upright or long sitting position, they are more than likely unable to achieve range due to a mobility dysfunction. To determine this, we can carry out further assessments and really hone in on what joint is affecting the rest.

I want to be clear: each joint has the ability to be both stable and mobile, as this is vital for basic movement functions. Joints are also, however, predisposed to favour either mobility or stability, in the same way our genetics predispose our muscle fibres to having faster or slower twitch orientation (think of Usain Bolt vs. a sumo wrestler). Joints with a predisposition towards stability include the midfoot, knee, lumbar spine, scapular and elbow. Conversely, the ankle, hip, shoulder and wrist favour the mobility side of our spectrum. I also want to be clear that this is an overview and not an all-inclusive list. The foot alone has 33 joints in it, and to break each of these down in terms of mobility vs. stability would be tedious. I am keeping this simple to get the point across. Joints coexist to give us both stability and mobility, creating our posture.

To determine whether the body is working in an organised fashion, we must view the individual's body as a whole. Filming their gait can achieve this. So can watching them pick up objects from the floor, reaching overhead and turning around. In the time it took me to write this, a number of assessments will have been carried out, some more effective than others to measure the ability and functionality of a person's joints to express stability and mobility.

I currently look at global movements, such as can a person touch their toes (or multi-segmental flexion), can they stand up and reach behind their head (multi-segmental extension), can they rotate symmetrically left and right through their neck (cervical spine), upper back (thoracic spine) and pelvis? Can this person squat, can they hinge, can they stand on one leg for a certain amount of time? These are objective measures that we can utilise to look at the interactions or lack of interactions between the major joints in their body. I will ask subjective questions about the pain they feel, how they feel their weight is distributed between their left and right legs in a standing position, and how they feel they distribute the weight on their pelvis in a seated position. Each person will be different, so do not rush through your assessments. We want to treat the person just as much, if not more so, than we want to treat their injury or movement deficiency. First, aim to understand the person. Do not fall into the trap of what I call 'pattern guessing' – an assumption that because we have seen a certain presentation before, all cases will be the same.

If you have not realised by now, our bodies are ingenious. We cannot apply the same treatment to each person. There may be similarities, but the difference lies in the amount of time since the injury occurred, the mechanism of injury and the person's action and perceived thoughts around themselves and their injury. The treatment plan should encompass all of this collected data.

Breathing has so far been neglected in all this talk about stability and mobility. Breathing is a form of both stability and mobility. I used an example in Chapter 1 where the response of someone stretching is to hold their breath as they try and force themselves into a new joint or muscle position – remember the tomato face? This, in my experience, has never improved their mobility or flexibility, at least not in the long term. We cannot have one part of the spectrum without the other.

Imagine an arc, as illustrated in Figure 4.1 below. We have a top, a middle and a bottom. If we start in the middle of our arc, we are the same distance away from the top as we are to the bottom. What if we are more predisposed to one end? Let's say I am at the top of the arc. I am a lot further away from the bottom now than I was when I was at the centre. This means I would have to travel a lot further to reach the bottom. We have these arcs within each joint in our body: a top and bottom, left and right, internal and external, pronation and supination. Whatever the name may be, the principle is the same. If I am out of position, favouring one side more than the other, it will be harder to access the side I am further away from.

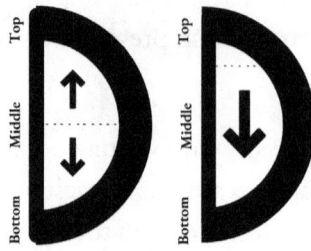

Figure 4.1

Our breath is a gateway to accessing the entirety of this arc of motion. If we do not breathe, we immediately inhibit our motion, supporting Gray Cook's statement of sacrificing mobility for stability. To create meaningful and lasting improvements within our spectrum between stability and mobility, breathing cannot be forgotten.

A big focus of my practice is to enable people to recapture this normal arc of their movement. First, we teach people using simple terms such as moving in and out, top, middle, bottom, etc.

Next, we assess them to figure out what they can and can't do and, more importantly, what the task they wish to do requires of them. How much input and movement do we need to change to enable them to reach their goal?

From here, we teach them how to use their joints by, for example, breaking down movement patterns before integrating them into larger motions, such as pelvic tilts and deadlifting. We also provide them with constraints to enable their body to easily fall into these positions.

The secret ingredient to all this is patience – you can't rush this process. You must learn to breathe through positions if you ever wish to own them. Once we have a novel understanding of all the internal movements, we can shift our centre of gravity accordingly. I shift their focus to an external environment. That is, having intent.

Think of attempting to pick up a bucket of water that you think will be heavy, and when you do it's light as a feather, easy. *Wow*, you think to yourself, *I thought that would be harder*. The physiological process behind this movement recruited more of your muscle, leading to a higher force output.

This is the end goal for movement: being able to exert force, intent and control through a pattern.

5

Learn Thy Principles

"No man has the right
to be an amateur in the
matter of physical training.
It is a shame for a man
to grow old without seeing
the beauty and strength of
which his body is capable."
- Socrates

The principles of training are the foundation of this book. Principles are absolute, numero uno, the top dog, the bee's knees – you get the drift. Principles are important within any effective training plan, business model, way of life. To create a training plan without abiding by the principles is careless. To some this can be limiting, for others, it is a source of endless creativity and methodologies to create effective and life-changing programmes. I implore you to choose the second way of thinking.

After a person has established their goals, encompassing a specific task to work towards, and once we understand their lifestyle, barriers and medical history, we can start to look towards building a programme.

A nifty acronym to remember the principles involved here is FITT: **F**requency, **I**ntensity, **T**ime and **T**ype of exercise.

FREQUENCY OF EXERCISE

This is measured by the number of days per week we dedicate to an exercise session. We must not overlook this first principle for a variety of reasons. The number of sessions we allocate towards our training programme can determine whether we successfully reach our goal. Too many and we overtrain, injure ourselves and wreak havoc on our neurological system. Too few and we undertrain, fail to provide enough impetus to keep going and become demotivated by a lack of results.

Like all concepts we have discussed thus far, there is a fine line between success and failure. The good news is that if you're new to training, you can get away with a lot less early on.

It's currently recommended that the ideal frequency of engagement with moderately to vigorously intense cardiovascular exercise is three to five sessions per week, or 150 minutes of moderately intense or 75 minutes of vigorously intense exercise.[26]

The ideal frequency will vary from person to person. Let me explain. In theory, it is easy to meet the targets outlined above for moderate to intense exercise every week. In practice, it's another kettle of fish. Life gets in the way – events, holidays, travel, work. There may be periods when we simply have very little free time. Is this to say we should just give up altogether and stop exercising? I strongly disagree. Make use of the time you have. If you can only commit to one or two sessions per week, this can still be more beneficial than not engaging in any movements whatsoever.

We know exercise is medicine; the research is unequivocal. Those that are sedentary are at a significantly greater risk of chronic disease and ill health. Some research does suggest that we should either engage in more than three sessions or not engage in any at all due to the risk of musculoskeletal injury. My view is that starting is better than nothing. Performing one session per week may be the initial catalyst you require to start the journey towards reaching your goals.

Through intelligent programming we can mitigate the risk of injury and still get benefits. Even if it's not optimal, we can still exercise less than the required amount to improve our nervous system economy, sleep, mood, mental health, balance and coordination, flexibility, body awareness, and that's just the start of the benefits. Yes, I implore you to consistently exercise, but don't be so hard on yourself if you can't. Some weeks, even just getting in a simple walk to clear your head may be what you need at that point in time.

When writing your programmes, aim for the desired intensities but take into account the individual's lifestyle. Do not ask someone who is available only two or three times per week to perform two sessions per day, every day. I have seen this happen far too often. Understand the person so you can work towards the recommendations gradually, and then they will prioritise their health rather than fear it.

INTENSITY

Just like any form of medicine, there is an optimal dosage. Exercise is no different. We mentioned that approximately 150 minutes of exercise spread over three to five sessions per week is the recommended frequency, but what about the type of exercise? Think of being prescribed 10mg of ibuprofen for a headache, but you only take 2.5mg – -it won't be as effective at alleviating your headache. Exercise is akin to this; we should strive for specific intensities in order to yield positive change.

Previously, we mentioned a range between 75 to 150 minutes per week, dependent on the level of intensity. The harder we work, the less we need to do, and vice versa.

So, what are these intensities and how do we know what they look like?

Low intensity is defined as using less than 50% of your maximum heart rate (HR). To identify our working HR, we can use the talk test.

This test basically measures how hard you are working when maintaining a conversation. If you can talk in full, complete sentences without needing to stop for breath, you're working at a relatively low intensity. Moderate intensity is between 50-85% of your maximum HR; you can still speak, but it's becoming harder to string a sentence together and you would rather focus on the task at hand.

Lastly, a vigorous intensity (85-100% of your maximum HR) is a huge struggle. I don't want to speak to you, I don't want to look at you, just leave me alone to wallow in my misery. We can't sustain this intensity for very long but, hey, luckily we don't have to before we reap the benefits.

This is a subjective way we can view our HR when we don't have access to fancy gadgets like a HR monitor or if we are taking medications that may influence our blood pressure and heart rate.

Intensity matters, so look to incorporate this so long as you can reap the benefits without underworking or overworking yourself. As a general guide, aim to sit within the moderate intensity of 70-85% of your maximum HR; this is often a sweet spot where you can get benefits without feeling like death while doing it.

TIME

Pretty straightforward this one. It's the amount of time we exercise during a given session, or the duration. We can get creative with how we allocate time for our sessions throughout the week.

If you only have three days a week to exercise at low-moderate intensity, you might take three 50-minute walks to make up your 150 minutes for the week. If you have more days free but less time on those days, you might walk 25 minutes on six days. The end result is the same. Match this with your lifestyle, and be sure it's something you can do consistently because, remember, a good programme is just words on paper if it's not completed. Too often we will shoot for the stars, get amped up with motivation and set an unrealistic target of every day, twice a day. Chances are if you don't have a regular habit of exercising, you won't stick to this one for long at all!

Another common alternative is breaking up your vigorous sessions throughout the day. Rather than doing it all in one big hit, you might do a short, high-intensity workout in the morning and then another session at night to accumulate your daily or weekly time. The possibilities with this are endless. There'll be something to suit everyone, so long as the individual is willing to prioritise their health enough.

TYPE

The type of exercises you perform should be specific to your goal. We cannot excel at activities in which we do not take part. Some movement patterns or skills are transferrable, but ultimately our physiological adaptations are specific to the type of exercise performed. My own bias and relationship with resistance-based training has enabled me to improve my physiological capabilities. This has transferred into movements and sports like running, soccer and athletics to enable me to generate more force, run more economically and become less injury prone due to my new sense of mobility and stability throughout my body. I could argue the need for some form of resistance training in people of all with various conditions and goals. Nonetheless, the take-home point is to make your activity specific to the goal at hand and what you're looking to achieve.

You now understand how you must 'FITT' these principles in with your goal. The FITT principles are a staple in all good programmes: use them to improve your health and create goal-orientated programmes that are individual to you.

Now, on to the heavy-hitting exercise prescription principles. Here lies the secret to creating evidence-based, effective programmes to yield the benefits of exercise training regardless of the modality you choose to pursue.

These principles are specificity, progressive overload, reversibility, adaptation and recovery.

SPECIFICITY

As mentioned, we become good at the tasks we perform. A quote from the late, great Bruce Lee comes to mind: "I fear not the man who practiced 10,000 kicks once, but I fear the man who has practiced one kick 10,000 times."

There's a reason they say practice makes perfect.

If want to play soccer competitively yet all you do is swim, what will be the result? Yes, you will improve your cardiovascular system and may be able to run around after the ball for longer, but it won't help your dribbling skills, your defending or your ability to score goals. Swimming will not help you meet the demands in soccer of running, jumping, kicking, heading, absorbing force, changing direction and balancing.

Be specific, break down what is required of the task and develop the skills directly.

PROGRESSIVE OVERLOAD

Who doesn't like progressing? Have you ever played a video game where a certain level or boss battle is really hard? What we often do in this instance is come back later when we are more equipped to handle it. Maybe we level up, or find new armour or weapons. Then, when faced with the same challenge, we can easily overcome the demands and move on to the next level or boss.

Apply this thinking to exercise. We engage with a certain type of exercise at a particular intensity, then next time we find it's easier. We have adapted. To continue this adaptation, we must gradually increase the difficulty.

Although we are talking about 'overload', I do not want you to fall into the trap of thinking this only applies to adding extra weight. This is not the case! We can progressively overload in a multitude of ways, ranging from decreasing our rest intervals, to performing more repetitions, to taking less time to complete a walk. You can focus on other variables while completing the same task. Someone new to training may find they progress by completing an extra session that week. Progressive overload comes in many forms. Be wise enough to take the time to look for progression in the mundane.

This principle must be followed if we are to prevent plateauing. If you have reached a plateau, then you've stopped adapting and I recommend looking at the variables of your training programme. This can broaden your horizons as you continue on your journey of discovery.

Look at your lifestyle and ask yourself questions like: are you sleeping enough (quantity) or having adequate rest (quality), eating a balanced diet, managing your hydration and stress levels? If you've answered no to any of the above, or any other questions you might have thought of, try working on those areas first. If this still has not changed anything and you are still at the plateau after two weeks, it is time to assess the effectiveness of your training programme and make modifications.

These modifications could come in the form of a selective decrease in intensity, maybe dropping from 10 sets to five for the week.

REVERSIBILITY

Have you ever heard the saying "use it or lose it"? This concept stems from reversibility. Our bodies are in a constant state of decline: we age, our reactions get slower, our muscles atrophy, we inevitably die – very morbid, I know.

The principle of reversibility opposes progressive overload; it's a constant reminder that we, as humans, will one day succumb and cease to exist. With progressive overload we improve with continued stressors; we adapt. It is only fair that without these stressors, if we become sedentary and stop or minimise the activity we once did, we decline, reversing the benefits gained through exercise.

This principle should be understood when writing training programmes to avoid or at least minimise its effects. During periods of high stress, work, or holidays, we can alter our training parameters to account for a drop in overload. This will enable us to stifle the ever-looming threat of reversibility and enable us to maintain rather than decline.

Longer periods of inactivity (more than six weeks) can often lead to significant drops in our ability to generate force, coordinate ourselves and use our cardiovascular system. Aim to move in some capacity daily, even if it's going for a walk around the block or standing up regularly from your chair at the office. Make movement a part of your day and minimise the effects of this principle.

ADAPTATION

Adaptation and progressive overload go hand in hand. In fact, adaptation is dependent upon progressive overload. We adapt to stimulus because our bodies are resilient. Think back to our antalgic gait: we change what we do and how we do it to avoid pain.

When we hit the sweet spot, or close to it, and apply the correct stimulus, our body will say, "Screw that, I don't want to go through that hell again." So, it improves. It improves its efficiency, it changes the constraints of our muscle fibres, tendons, bones and nervous system to overcome the stimulus in case it has to face it again. Adaptation is a form of survival, a biological advantage to overcome our environment. To adapt, our bodies need a challenge, time to recover and then a new challenge. This simple cycle is how our body improves over time.

RECOVERY

We spend approximately one-third of our life sleeping (based on the recommended eight hours per day). Knowing this, I guess we could say recovery is worth talking about. We need to prioritise recovery after the application of stimulus (overload) in order to adapt or even just to perform again.

Think of this like wiping up some liquid you spilt on the floor. You wipe the liquid with a sponge, only there's still more, so you'll have to rinse the sponge and repeat until you soak up all the spilt liquid. This process of rinse and repeat is akin to you hitting your capacity. You can only take in so much stimulus before you need to rest. Only then can you go back and do more.

If we don't recover adequately, our body can suffer from overuse injuries, psychological and physical exhaustion and a lack of healing. Recovery is a crucial component when getting the dosage of exercise correct. With adequate recovery we can achieve incredible feats; without it, we become zombies – lifeless, slow and brain-dead.

How do we know we have recovered?

Let's say you went to a gym on a Monday and performed a lower-body workout. You want to train your legs twice a week, so you plan on going on Thursday but your legs are still really sore from your first workout on Monday. Have you recovered? No, not completely.

Before commencing training again, we must let our body recuperate for several reasons. Muscle damage is not a necessary factor for muscle growth; sore muscles can inhibit strength, cause stiffness and lead to mild discomfort. This has negative implications for your upcoming training session because it will impede your ability to perform. If you go into your sessions with a low intensity when you should be aiming for a moderate to high intensity, the benefits from the session will be minimal. Don't be afraid to alter your session. There are other ways you can stay active during periods of recovery, such as swimming, walking, cycling and gentle stretches.

Then, maybe you're feeling like a million dollars again by Friday and you can complete your session with decent enough intensity to elicit good stimulus for you to adapt. Woohoo!

EXERCISE SELECTION

Exercise selection is not necessarily a principle, but more of a consideration in the art of programming. When picking an exercise, we want to determine if the selected movement is appropriate for us. Ask yourself the following questions:

1. What is my level of training?

2. Have I done this specific movement/exercise before?

3. Do I have any injuries that need to be accounted for?

4. Does this exercise help me move towards my goal?

5. Is this a progression of a previous movement?

Basically, we want a solid rationale for our exercise selection. If we are doing burpees just to make a session hard, we are missing the point. Our exercises should be focused on quality rather than quantity. We are not just trying to fill time; we are trying to cultivate healthy biomechanical patterns through targeted exercise.

Don't be afraid to seek guidance if you're unsure of an exercise or movement. Some of you will be able to break down the skill yourself before building it up into the proper movement, others may need added assistance through a coach or trainer – we can't all be proprioceptive genii!

While exercise is regarded as medicine, too much of something can be a bad thing. In this case, the inappropriate dosage or type of exercise can lead to injury, trauma and fear avoidance. We can create almost as many issues through unstructured movements. That is why I am writing this book, to give you the tools required to engage in programmes and empower yourself!

Exercise Selection based on Type

Our exercise selection can alter drastically depending on what an individual wants. If someone wants to lose weight, they may have a programme revolving around large, multi-joint, compound movements which expend a lot of energy. These involve large ranges of motion with multiple muscles. If I was to give you the choice between a bicep curl and a deadlift for losing weight, what would you choose? (*cough, deadlift, cough, cough*).

If we are looking at someone wishing to gain significant muscle mass (hypertrophy focus), we will incorporate large multi-joint muscles as well as isolation-based exercises. This will enable sufficient stimulus to occur within our intended area of growth.

If we are in a rehabilitation setting, we would look to incorporate low threshold movements, aimed at developing a structural base to work from. The exercises would be both localised and global to help the person regain a sense of their lost range of motion, strength and proprioception (body awareness). Exercise selection should always have a purpose. Again, this is not a principle but I would argue it should be.

Ok, ready to put this together?

We have Betsy. Betsy is a middle-aged woman, with no medical conditions or complications. Betsy has had a shoulder injury in the past which can still be aggravated if she pushes herself too hard. Betsy is new to exercise and wants to improve her body composition. Betsy has tried weight-training classes in the past and enjoyed the variety. Betsy gets bored walking so prefers not to do this unless she has to. Betsy is also hesitant about performing really hard sessions and explained that classes becoming too difficult was why she stopped exercising in the first place. Betsy has said she can only commit to around 80 minutes of exercise per week due to work commitments, driving her children around and doing volunteer work in the evenings.

Let's break this example down. Betsy has an unspecific goal of losing some weight; for argument's sake, let's say 5kg to give us some more context. Betsy can commit to about 80 minutes of exercise per week – this puts her in the category of moderate-vigorous exercise if we want her to hit the recommended physical activity guidelines straight away. Betsy is also a novice, so putting her through some pretty rough training may not be ideal at the moment. So, what do we do?

Utilising the FITT principles, we want Betsy performing three or four sessions per week. The intensity will fluctuate between low to moderate and moderate to vigorous. Each exercise activity will be around 20 to 25 minutes based on her availability of roughly 80 minutes per week. Betsy has previously engaged in weight-based training which she enjoyed, but also has a shoulder injury. Ideally, she'll need to perform large compound whole-body movements for the weight loss, but it's also worth performing unilateral or single-arm movements for her injured shoulder. Now, Betsy isn't a fan of walking as structured exercise so we can look at alternatives like cycling to supplement her weight training.

A programme can come in many different shapes and forms and will largely depend on the person. This programme is suitable for Betsy as it matches both the criteria and her lifestyle. It will be an effective way for Betsy to reach her goal of losing weight and avoid aggravating her shoulder. I hope this has sparked your creativity. Now we have broken down the principles behind writing a training programme, you can feel free to play around and create a million ways for Betsy to reach her objective or start mapping out your own!

6

Motion Is Lotion

"A pattern is either right
or wrong...it is no stronger
than its weakest point."
-William Morris

P atterns exist in everything we do. The way we write, the
way we walk, our morning routine, the way we drive. We
are but a collection of patterns. Within these movement patterns
are large segmental motions using a range of joints, angles and
structures that we carry out every day to complete tasks.

Each person has developed a particular biomechanical structure
– the shape of your bones, your muscles, your tendons, and how
they attach to other structures within your body, the way they
work together to create joint angles which enable us to move. We
covered patterns that exist within the human gait: cycle, flexion,
extension, internal and external rotation to name a few. When
carrying out everyday tasks, like picking up clothes from the
floor, reaching overhead, carrying groceries and so on, we use
our bodies in different ways to create patterns. We require these
patterns because they give us the movement to access, utilise
and dominate the activities of our daily living with relative ease.

These patterns are trainable; we can strengthen or weaken them through guided or imbalanced exercise regimes.

There are six basic areas of human movement: hinging, squatting, pulling, pushing, carrying and our gait (which we covered previously). We rely on each of these patterns every day, consciously and unconsciously. We may be bias to certain patterns more than others, which can be due to demographics (different cultures and lifestyles), exposure to specific styles of training or sports, muscle imbalances and a host of other reasons.

If we compare Eastern and Western cultures, there are a number of key differences that can dictate or at least influence the way we develop and utilise patterns within our everyday movements. In Western cultures, people predominantly sit on chairs and sleep on elevated beds. We are often fixed at 90-degree angles, whether sitting at a desk, table or on the toilet to name a few. In contrast, people in Eastern cultures will often adopt a more ground-based approach, having legless chairs or pillows, squatting rather than sitting and the like.

What implications does this have for us? This is where the SAID principle comes into play, which states our body will have specific adaptation to our imposed demands, meaning it will adapt to our environment.

Let's look at the pattern used when squatting. In Eastern cultures, people generally have large degrees of hip flexion and ankle dorsiflexion, a full range of motion, in other words, which allows them to maintain this pattern with relative ease. Westerners, however, are biased towards a pattern of poor squatting. The ankle and hip ranges of flexion and extension become somewhat limited due to being fixed at 90 degrees frequently. It should be noted this is a massive generalisation. I am aware that people of both cultures can and do engage in a range of sitting and sleeping positions. I am merely stating that the environment of each culture promotes key differences that can mean the body favours certain patterns. I have worked with individuals of Eastern backgrounds who couldn't squat to save their life and people of Western backgrounds who look like they invented the squat. Nevertheless, if we place ourselves within an environment that isn't suitable for the task, we can become bias towards a pattern of poor squatting. The ankle and hip ranges of flexion and extension become somewhat limited. Irrespective of your background, I want you to understand the impact of your immediate environment and how you can use or alter specific movements when carrying out daily activities to reach targeted outcomes.

The style of training you engage with can leave you either mobile or immobile. As I have previously mentioned, in the case of powerlifters, we can become exceptional at areas such as a sagittal plane or forward and backwards actions, and neglect other planes of transverse and frontal, which in turn will lead to an inability to move freely. Be aware of the style of your training. Much like sitting in a certain position throughout your life can affect your range of motion, you can bet that training particular patterns, over and over, while neglecting others can also change what we can and cannot access within our bodies. The exercises and movements we usually hate to perform are often the ones we need the most. They are hard because we are using other patterns, planes or positions that we have not yet mastered. Assess your own bias, find out what you need, and what you currently have and go from there to create programmes that encourage healthy, controlled movements rather than limiting stifling ones.

Lastly, bias towards particular patterns can occur through muscle imbalances, structural deficits, injury and the like. If I have injured my ankle, I may predispose myself towards patterns of hinging where a large degree of movement in the ankle is not required like it would be if I was to squat. Maybe again through the way I have trained, I have developed muscle imbalances and become exceptionally strong in pushing actions, but not so much in pulling. Now I will be biased toward a range that allows my muscles to go one way, but not necessarily the other. I may even have a genetic birth defect that inhibits me from loading myself proportionately due to limb imbalances. Injury can cause us to adopt antalgic patterns, ones that offload and prevent the painful stimulus from occurring. If uncorrected, we will have developed a new pattern; the question is if this is sustainable in the long term. The way we move is dictated by our bones, muscles and nervous system. These are developed in utero, in early childhood and then throughout the rest of our lives to maintain, grow or atrophy.

THE BIRDS AND THE BEES

Have you ever thought about how we learn to move in the early stages of life?

When two people love each other very much they ... ok, too far back?

Early learning may look like mastering how to roll over, stand up from the floor and start walking. Have you ever watched a young child figure out how to complete the above tasks?

Developmental kinesiology refers to the patterns we develop as infants to allow us to move. Basically, from birth we need to figure out how to move our body, stand up and get to the food we crave. This is a well-documented area, one that allows us to view the development of our patterns through our early life, namely within the first 21 months. We have a distinct timeline for exactly when we should be accomplishing a range of patterns, and this enables us to step in to correct errors or delays along the learning curve of movement proficiency.

At the time of writing this, I am of the strong belief that developmental kinesiology, the healthy growth of fundamental patterns, dictates how we grow and how we move later in life. It's much like how our childhood and the associated trauma or lack thereof can dictate our future and how we perceive and act in the world around us. This is a well-researched and agreed-upon concept in psychosocial and behavioural studies.

I have seen a number of people that have been exposed to what I deem 'excessive' stability at young ages without having learned how to stabilise themselves through the good ol' 'fall down and get back up' trick. This excessive stability comes in the form of ambulation aids such as bouncers and walkers, or parents carrying their children and forcing them into these positions before they are required, or have earnt the right to access them.

Why is this a problem? Remember the SAID principle and antalgic gait. We develop around what we have. If we learn to use the incorrect muscles to stabilise, we will break our imaginary chain of segmental joints and muscle recruitment and develop a host of compensations when forming our basic movement patterns. Later in life, this can look like overpronated or supinated feet, chronic hip tightness, knee valgus, hip hikes or rotations. These are just some of the issues that can arise in the lower body, not to mention the upper body. Yet, life does go on. It isn't all doom and gloom. If you are exposed to a certain way of doing things from birth, you will adapt to it. It may not be the most efficient and effective way, but it'll still work.

Developmental kinesiology represents a natural order, and within this early stage of life our central nervous system and primitive reflexes develop the ability to adopt a low level of trunk stability. This is essential for coordinating locomotion of the extremities and normal respiration; without it we become inefficient lumps of mass.[27] Some of the concepts within the systems of dynamic neuromuscular stabilisation (DNS), functional movement screens (FMS) and the postural restoration institute (PRI) can be used to illustrate our progression through movement stages. Throughout our life we are able to create more complex and larger movement patterns at fundamental, transitional and functional levels.

Fundamental Level – Supine, Prone, Rolling, Quadruped and Crawling.

Transitional Level – Sitting, kneeling and squatting.

Functional Level – Standing up and walking.

The development of our movement in early childhood is illustrated in the image above. In an ideal world, we pass through each stage as and when we earn the right, leading to healthy, orchestrated and controlled movement patterns. These patterns are ancient and exist within us at a cellular level, or at least have the potential to exist within all humans. They are shaped by our bone structure, our muscle origins and insertions, and our physiology. Without these patterns, movement as we know it ceases to exist. The human race cannot procreate and pass on its genes to the next generation and we become extinct. Now, do you understand why movement patterns are essential and should not be overlooked?

I understand the gravity of the above statement: that if we can't get some basic movements under wraps, we won't be able to procreate. Bit of a stretch, I know. Nonetheless, at least you are now aware of the importance of movement and transitional levels. If you want to be a badass human that works in three planes of dimension and is a fully functional, well-lubricated specimen, capable of beautiful, synergistic movement with access to everything you want and need, then you need to start with movement patterns.

Developmental kinesiology can be a viable place to start with people that have lost their movement capabilities. It can bridge the gap between stability and mobility to allow them to realign with their primitive selves, the ones that allowed them to move in the first place. These exercises are typically low-level movements. You cannot force your way through them, rather patience and control of the small intricacies is required. Through this, you develop proprioception – body awareness – and harness the ability to organise your body in a segmental flow once again.

PRIMAL PATTERNS

Once we have learned the fundamental levels of laying, rolling and crawling, we look to take on the world through standing, squatting and walking.

So, what comes next?

Enter the primal patterns: our large, multi-joint movements that have dominated the health and fitness world. When programming for healthy movement, we want to ensure we use the majority if not all of the primal patterns, or at least know how to access them for exceptional quality movement.

I want you to get up and perform a simple task. Put a nearby object on the floor and pick it up.

What did you notice? Did you squat (bend your ankle, knee and hips) or hinge (push your bum back) to pick up the object?

You will have wired your neurons to act unconsciously when performing this pattern of movement. We train them to be biased towards one pattern and completely neglect the alternative, leading to limitations in our movement capabilities. Knowing our biases, strengths, weaknesses and patterns goes a long way to improving our movement quality.

The fundamental movements that each person requires for a decent range include pulling, pushing, carrying squatting, hinging and gait.

These patterns are the crux of human life and motion. How we combine them is the key to healthy movement.

I am aware of the many differences that exist within movement patterns. However, the six patterns serve as a guideline for general programming advice applicable to everyone. The patterns of walking have been covered in previous chapters and lunging and crawling are what I consider subcomponents of the larger patterns.

PUSHING

The pattern of pushing encompasses all planes of motion. The sagittal, transverse and frontal can be accessed in movements such as bench presses, woodchops, lunges and crab walking to name a few. These patterns are commonly used within gym settings as both a horizontal and vertical axis movement. Push-ups are an example of the horizontal axis, while shoulder pressing is an example of the vertical axis. Everyday acts of pushing could be moving a shopping trolley, closing the fridge and mowing the lawn.

When I say pushing, I want you to understand that this pattern is everywhere. We can even call squatting a version of pushing. Pushing is expansion. Taking us back to the breath briefly, we can view pushing as an outward force away from us, i.e., the exhalation.

PULLING

Pulling, like pushing, is an essential part of life. In contrast to our pushing patterns, we can view pulling as compression, the drawing in or inhalation of our breath. Common movements that train the pulling patterns include deadlifting (I consider this a pushing movement to an extent as well), rowing, lat pulldowns, leg curls and the like. Everyday movements may be pulling a door open, opening a drawer or pulling a shopping trolley out of a row of trolleys.

To have balance within our training, we must have a healthy balance of pushing and pulling, much like we must have a balanced breath – too much emphasis on one part can lead to compensation on the opposing side.

CARRYING

As bipeds, we humans have the ability to carry objects of various shapes and sizes and walk at the same time. This is a huge pattern for us as a species overall. It enables the quick transportation of objects, and multi-tasking and ultimately helps us to survive. It's one of the key skills that has contributed to the advancement of humankind.

You've hunted and killed your prey. It's dead, so you have a meal and can live another day. Only, your wife and children are many miles away as you had to run after this animal to kill it. What can you do?

Option A) Ignore your family, have a feast and watch the human race die out.

Option B) You can carry the kill back to your family/tribe and feed them as well, ensuring the survival of your species.

Carrying does not have quite the same dramatic consequences these days. Our inability to carry or even lift up an object properly can lead to time off work or missing out on recreational activities due to injury. It can lead to chronic pain, compensation and rapid fatigue. Learning the art of carrying is an important step for an individual wishing to access and own their body's full spectrum of movement. In a gym this can be zercher squats, dead hangs and deadlifts, while in everyday life it can be walking with a suitcase, carrying the groceries inside or emptying your bins.

SQUATTING

The squat is one of the most well-known movements; think of sitting down on a chair. This can be done exceptionally well when well-practised or very poorly by those unacclimatised to this important skill.

Squatting is, in essence, a push of the lower body; as we extend our legs upwards and move our body away from the floor, we are pushing. We've all seen the signs explaining that the correct way to lift something is to "bend your knees instead of your back", even though this has recently been shown to be poor advice (you can lift more weight with a curved back!). The squat is a versatile and functional movement.

We need to squat. It has been a common pattern throughout generations when cooking, cleaning, communicating and going to the toilet. Eastern cultures have maintained this. Our physiology is designed for a deep squat, as opposed to planting ourselves at a 90-degree angle. Our colons are a prime example of this. If we squat completely, ass to grass or whatever you wish to call it, we give our colon a direct passage from which to pass faeces. Think of bending a water hose vs. keeping it unkinked; the difference in fluid pressure and flow is significant. Children are great to watch as they illustrate freedom of movement. They will often either squat or hinge.

You are the same. When I asked you to try and pick something up like you normally would, you should have found you will either squat or bend over (hinge). Children have not been yet moulded and fixed into these unnatural positions, such as sitting at 90 degrees, and will often fully realise their mobility potential: they will perform an ass-to-grass squat with relative ease, almost like they are autonomous in the art of squatting. The squat is considered an anterior chain pattern (front side of our body).

Hinging

Hinging is a favourite pattern of mine to teach. As a coach, I find this is probably one of the most difficult patterns to grasp for most people, especially for those that have chronic pain — back and hip pain in particular. Why? you ask. Well, it requires segmental control. A large part of these segments is made up of your thoracolumbar column and your pelvis, in other words, your trunk. It involves shifting weight, and a delicate balance so we don't fall backwards or forwards. Instead, we are like tightrope walkers, adjusting multiple joints in unison to accomplish a biomechanical feat. The hinge exists within everyday actions, such as picking objects off the floor, leaning over, bowing and playing golf. The hinge is the amalgamation of pulling and carrying.

We will see this when deadlifting, swinging kettlebells or performing 'good mornings' at the gym. It allows us to target our posterior chain (back side of us from ankle to head) and develop serious power and strength for moving forward. Jumping, running and the like require our posterior chain, which we can target using the hinge pattern to make us more athletic.

Knowing these movements is the first step towards becoming a badass human. The next step is knowing how and when to apply them, and what to do if we struggle with a particular pattern. We will cover this later on.

Slings

While not patterns per se, our slings are worth mentioning as vital parts of coordinating and creating movement. We have many, but two key slings are worth highlighting: the anterior oblique sling (AOS) and the posterior oblique sling (POS). The synergy of these slings is a key driver for human movement: think crawling, walking, stepping, running, swimming and throwing. These all rely on our slings. Slings work through reciprocal patterns, that is, opposites. Take gait (walking): we swing our left arm forward, and our right arm pulls back. Our left leg goes forward, our right leg is back. If we cut your body in two equal halves, we would have one side pushing and one side pulling to allow us to move. This, in essence, is your body rotating and counterrotating to enable your freedom of movement. The anterior oblique sling comprises of muscles like the internal and external obliques of the stomach, and the adductor (inner thigh) on the opposing leg.

The posterior oblique sling, as the name implies, refers to the back side of us, muscles such as the latissimus dorsi, gluteus maximus (bum) and biceps femoris (hamstring) to name a few. They work together to create a posterior sling.

The opposing or contralateral limbs will often work together, These are hardwired into us so we can accelerate, decelerate and maintain stability within our torso as we undertake locomotion. Watch yourself next time you walk or run or swim. Your opposing limbs will naturally (if you haven't developed compensations) swing in unison. This may look like stepping forward with your right leg, and your left arm swings forward as well. Both our AOS and POS are at play here, battling for predominance as we shift through the cycle of motion.

The intricacies of human movement could occupy a thousand more books. I have briefly touched on each concept here to make you aware of these concepts. Now I implore you to continue reading multiple sources, using whatever style of learning suits you so you can understand and utilise these patterns. This will improve your life by fulfilling the potential of movement that exists within all of us.

7

Creating a Mona Lisa

"Art and science have their meeting point in method."
- Edward G. Bulwer-Lytton

We have a basic understanding of the training principles, but how do we now apply them? How do we create programmes that abide by these principles and still encourage creativity? The answer lies in the methods we use.

While the principles do not change, the methods do. There are a variety of ways to adhere to the principles of progressive overload, specificity, recovery, adaptation and exercise selection. There are unlimited training methodologies which can be used to create both simple and sophisticated programming.

The variables that we have not yet discussed include repetitions, sets, tempo, rest, format and order of the workout. Plus we can look at volume and intensity in greater depth.

REPETITIONS

Repetitions, or reps, refers to the number of times you perform an exercise, e.g., swimming five laps of a pool or lifting a weight 10 times in a row. It is a collection of repeated actions to complete a certain movement.

We can use reps as a tool for tracking progress, as a guide for intensity and as a target during our exercise programmes. The reps can vary drastically within a programme to achieve specific outcomes.

Want to develop strength? We may put you on the lower side of repetitions, such as less than five for a set.

Want to learn a new movement pattern? We need repetition, so we will aim for more reps.

Want to measure if you are getting stronger or adapting to a certain weight or stimulus? We can track how many repetitions you can complete at the given task over a period of time. You can see how we can use this variable to manipulate the constructs of our training programmes to reach our predetermined goal.

SETS

Sets are made up of a certain number of reps for a given exercise. Using the above example, if I wanted to swim five laps (reps) then rest, and repeat this again, I have completed two sets. So, your written programme would look something like 'two (sets) of five (reps)' for that particular exercise.

Just like reps, we can manipulate the number of sets we perform to achieve certain goals. Sets will be directly impacted by your training age. If you are a novice beginning your first exercise programme, we can get away with fewer sets to reap the benefits of exercise. As we progress our training towards becoming our advanced archetype, we will need a greater stimulus to attain continued benefits from exercising. This may look like a novice completing one set of 10 repetitions compared to an intermediate trainer completing three sets of 10 repetitions and an advanced individual completing five sets of 10 repetitions. The variables of sets and reps combine to make up another essential training variable called volume.

VOLUME

Training volume refers to the amount of work we do for a particular exercise, i.e., the number of sets and reps. If we had someone perform three sets of 10 repetitions, their volume for that exercise is 30 reps. Let's say the exercise for this is lifting a weight of 10kg. We can calculate the volume for this exercise by multiplying three (sets) x 10 (reps) x 10 (kg) to give us 300kg lifted. Sounds like a lot, doesn't it? Who wouldn't prefer to say they lifted 300kg rather than 10kg?

Volume is crucial for progression and a very strong predictor for all of the principles of training. We can use volume to our advantage to enhance certain parameters of overload, adaptation, recovery and reversibility. If we apply volume to progressive overload, we can determine the volume required to achieve a particular result. If we are talking about the process of hypertrophy (gaining muscle), we can measure the volume required to make progress. For example, let's say I am required to complete 10 sets of chest exercises per week to see improvements with this muscle over time. If I complete less than, say, six sets per week, I may not create enough stimulus for adaptation or hypertrophy of the muscle. If I complete 14 sets per week, I may not recover well enough and overreach/overtrain, leading to reversibility in results. Getting the balance right when it comes to volume can be a bit hit-and-miss when first writing a programme. I would stay on the side of undertraining a person with less volume than overtraining them with too much. It is a much simpler process to add volume to someone's training load rather than undoing the negative effects associated with overtraining.

INTENSITY

Intensity, as a FITT principle, refers to the amount of effort we apply to an activity. We can measure intensity through a range of tools, such as our rate of perceived exertion (RPE) and repetitions in reserve (RIR) which are based on how hard we deem an activity and our heart rate percentage. These tools allow us to scale and measure the difficulty of our training thresholds. Intensity and volume are interdependent, which means that volume reduces as intensity increases or vice versa.

A bodyweight squat for 10 repetitions is a low-intensity workout for most people, meaning you could probably do this with ease. But if I added 50kg to your back and asked you to do it again, you may find this more difficult and struggle to get to the 10th repetition. If I doubled the weight on your back to 100kg and asked you to squat again, you may only manage five repetitions. As the task becomes more difficult, the number of times we can repeat it decreases. This applies to all movements. As we have already discussed, when it comes to FITT principles, we can attain the same benefits when doing exercises at either lower or higher intensities; the difference comes in the amount of time we must commit to them.

Remember, moderate to vigorous intensities require only 75 minutes of physical activity per week compared to low to moderate intensities requiring 150 minutes of physical activity per week.

TEMPO

Tempo of movement is another variable we can alter. It refers to the speed at which we control the repetition, which we can measure through the entirety of the rep: the starting point of the movement, the amount of time it takes to lift the weight up (concentric), the time of pause at the top and then the lowering down of the weight (eccentric).

In the context of a gym, the tempo is measured using four numbers. A common format you will see is: 3010. Let's use the example of a squat and match it to this tempo.

As we lower down to a squat position, our muscle is lengthening. This is called the eccentric phase, which corresponds with the first number you see above, 3, meaning we lower ourselves down for three seconds. The second number, 0, indicates how long we stay at the bottom of our squat. In this case, we don't spend any time there and stand straight back up. This brings us to the concentric phase, when we shorten our muscle. The third number, 1, means we have one second to get back to our starting position. The final number, 0, is the amount of time we spend at the top of our squat before commencing our next repetition. Now, if our set of squats involves 10 repetitions, that's approximately four seconds per repetition, or 40 seconds per set if we were strict with our tempo guidelines.

In the context of other sports and physical activities, like running, we may look at tempo in terms of the speed or cadence at which our feet hit the ground. There are many ways to track tempo and speed, and they will differ slightly from exercise to exercise. This is a malleable variable that we can use to determine the intensity at which we perform. If you are short on time and want a hard workout, you can perform a few exercises back-to-back with, say, 10 seconds of rest in between each. If you had more time and were looking to strength train, you might have two to three minutes of rest between each set of exercises. The exercises are the same, but the programme and the outcomes are entirely different.

Rest

Our rest periods enable us to increase the intensity with ease. They will be different depending on the style of training. Let's use the example of a walk. This is a low-intensity exercise. So, if I asked you to walk 100m at a certain speed, then stop briefly, and repeat, this would be an easy task because of the low level of movement required. However, if we changed it from a walk to a sprint, could you do it at the same pace, again and again? The short answer is no. We require a much longer rest period to achieve the same output as we did in our first 100m sprint. Why is this? you ask. Good question!

We have a number of energy systems within our body, and each one needs different rest periods depending on what we are trying to achieve.

The state of energy

In my first draft of this section, I waxed lyrical about an outdated principle. Luckily, the publishing process is slow! Since then, I have learnt about a new paradigm of energy. I credit Sean Seale and Evan Peikon, prominent professionals in the health and fitness industry, for educating me about this model. I'll now do my best to pass on what i've learnt.

Our three energy systems are called ATP-CP, or 'alactic', anaerobic or 'lactic' and aerobic. Each one is predominant at ALL times within the context of physical activity. It was previously thought that one system would be dominant over the others at certain times, leaving them largely redundant. But thanks to technological advances, researchers are now able to measure each system in greater depth, including exactly when they initiate. It is now apparent that the anaerobic and aerobic systems work in unison, albeit at varying degrees and times throughout exercise.

Previously, it was thought that the aerobic system took a back seat during the first 10 seconds of movement in, say, a 100m sprint. Now we realise that the biochemical relationship between oxygen and phosphocreatine is tightly coupled – meaning we cannot have one without the other.

Our body's systems for managing energy are the same as its systems for controlling movement — they are all connected!

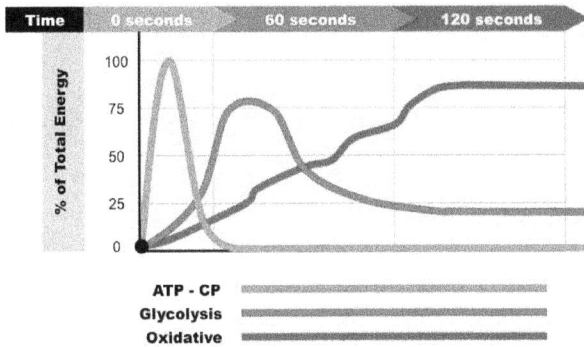

Figure 7.1

This model illustrates the old way of thinking, as mentioned – each system peaks and falls over a short time span, with the aerobic system being the predominant means of energy production after around 60 seconds of continuous movement.

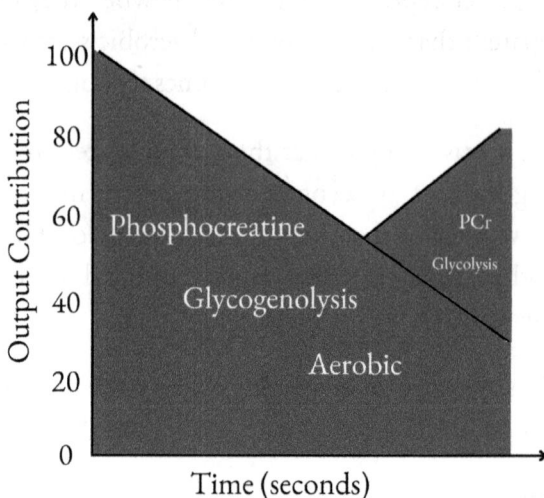

Figure 7.2 – Source: Aaron Davis

Bare with me in the following paragraph as this may become quite technical.

Figure 7.2 illustrates the new paradigm. Why is this relevant though? Well, one reason pertains to muscle contractions and how we utilise energy throughout our body to move. To contract a muscle, we rely on the body's energy currency, which is adenosine triphosphate (ATP), which breaks down into adenosine diphosphate (ADP). The role of the energy cycles shown in Figure 7.2 is to recycle the ADP and turn it back into ATP for further energy. [28] The old system (Figure 7.1) becomes outdated as advances in technology have occurred. Phosphocreatine (PCr) is the quickest form of regeneration of ATP which was previously assumed to occur without the presence of oxygen (O2). It is now apparent that oxygen (O2) is required to replenish PCr.[29] Keep in mind, that the harder we work (intensity) during exercise, the more oxygen we utilise. Now ATP is broken down extremely quick in the body between 10-40 milliseconds (ms). Once broken down, PCr will resynthesis ATP from ADP within 15 ms. Following this, a process called glycogenolysis occurs where our bodies use glycogen (carbohydrates that have been stored in our liver and muscles) to aid the recycling process of

ATP. [30] During this process Lactate is produced, which provides more of that wonderful ATP to our body.

Lactate was previously the villain of this story as being the mechanism of the burning sensation in your muscles after a hard bout of exercise. This is no longer the case. Recent research shows that lactate is always present in the body and helps fuel your energy systems, at rest, during work or while you're sitting there reading this book. Lactate is being produced. You can recycle this faster than the rate of accumulation leading you to not notice it at lower intensities. [31] This is where the final main system — the aerobic system comes in. Once glycogen is broken down it becomes glucose. To stay active, our bodies must recycle this glucose back into glycogen for further use. There will come a point where your O2 levels will decrease due to sustained exercise. You now won't be able to keep up with the above processes and you will eventually run out of ATP aka energy.

WHAT SHOULD YOU TAKE FROM ALL THIS?

- The body is a big recycling system. If the rate that rubbish accumulates exceeds the body's ability to recycle the rubbish then we have a breakdown or stop being able to perform at the level we require.

- There are no anaerobic athletes or aerobic athletes. Everyone is both, as O2 and Lactate are always required during physical activity or at rest.

- People will use their ATP in varying degrees based on the demands required of them. E.g., Sprinters will empty their so-called tank quicker than an aerobic athlete, who will aim to keep it as full as possible.

- Energy systems are ultimately limited by a person's respiratory system, not their anaerobic/lactic ability. In other words, oxygen drives performance.

- Different people will be limited by different measures.

The above point refers to three main areas or archetypes that people can be limited. Their utilisation ability, their delivery ability and/ or their respiratory ability. Think of this in the following way:

Utilisation limitation = Muscle

Delivery limitation = Heart

Respiration limitation = Lungs

If you've never trained, you may have a utilisation issue from a lack of muscle. If you've trained and have the muscle mass you may have a delivery limitation as your heart can't pump enough oxygen to those muscles. Lastly, if you have really good utilisation ability and a strong heart, an athlete such as a cyclist may be limited in their ability to exchange gas e.g. oxygen in and carbon dioxide out. The point I want you to take away from all of this is to have a basic understanding of the energy pathways and what your chosen activity requires. This can lead to changes in nutrition, training intensities, frequencies and how we structure our training regime as a whole.

FORMAT

You can get really creative with the formatting of your programme. We can use countless variations to target certain muscles, aim for specific outcomes, expose weaknesses, develop tenacity and engage ourselves with a multitude of scenarios. The format refers to how we structure our exercises within any given workout. This will vary from person to person, depending on their goals, skill level and availability.

It is well known that what we train first, we train best. This is common sense, but it also holds true from a physiological perspective based on the principles of rest and recovery. It's only natural that we will tire after a given period of exercising, leading to a drop in intensity or ability to exert output at a specific level until we rest and recover. Have you ever tried to cram a million activities into your day? This might start off well; you're attentive and bouncing with energy from activity to activity. But as the day lingers so does your energy. You start slowing down, talking less, thinking about sleep more and more. This is fatigue.

We can format our programme to prioritise particular activities to ensure we get the most out of them. For example, if my goal is to enhance a specific area of my body like my arms, I'd start my workout with bicep curls and triceps extensions to ensure I can generate sufficient intensities to create adaptation. This follows the principle of specificity: prioritising specific movements to achieve our task.

Now, let's look at potential formats we may use depending on the adaptation we are after. These will mostly apply to a gym-based setting, however, do not let this deter you from understanding the main point that formats allow us to be creative with how we engage with exercises, whatever they might be.

Each example below includes a table in which you will see that the sets, reps and tempo are the same. The difference is in the format: how the exercises are paired and the rest periods. This will hopefully help you keep track of the endless variables at play.

STRAIGHT SETS

A straight set is one of the simplest programme formats. We perform one exercise followed by a rest period of whatever time we allocate. This is a great way to focus on a specific exercise, allowing us to grow in technique with relatively little fatigue. The downfall of this style is it can be time-consuming if we were to perform three or four sets per exercise. I would still recommend that a novice starts with straight sets when exercising, as they can focus more on the technique rather than the psychological aspects of pushing through multiple sets in a row. This is also ideal for a newbie because adaptation can be gained with low volume.

Exercise	Sets	Reps	Rest	Tempo
1. Squat	3	10-12R	60s	3010
2. DB Press	3	10-12R	60s	3010
3. KB Deadlift	3	10-12R	60s	3010
4. DB Row	3	10-12R	60s	3010

Figure 7.3

SUPERSETS

Super sets are one of the most common formats for a gym programme. The pairing of two movements together creates a superset. This may look like performing one set, having a quick break or no rest at all and then engaging in another exercise before having our extended rest period. This is an incredible way to elicit a high amount of stimulus within a short amount of time.

You can change the variations of lower and upper exercises (more on this soon). Generally, this will favour people looking to grow muscle (hypertrophy), but it's still useful for all demographics.

Exercise	Sets	Reps	Rest	Tempo
A1. Squat A2. DB Press	3	10-12R	60s	3010
B1. KB Deadlift B2. DB Row	3	10-12R	60s	3010

Figure 7.4

TRI-SETS

Three movements together form a tri-set. This is an effective way of creating densely-packed workouts, exposing the individual to multiple movements across their workout so they can impact a large number of areas in a short amount of time.

Exercise	Sets	Reps	Rest	Tempo
A1. Squat A2. DB Press A3. Farmers Carry	3	10-12R	60s	3010
B1. KB Deadlift B2. DB Row B3. Calf Raise	3	10-12R	60s	3010

Figure 7.5

GIANT SETS

This is like a fast or miniature circuit. With this style, we combine four exercises together before our much-needed rest period. These can be a mixture of upper and lower body or just all lower body or upper body movements. The possibilities really are endless. Giant sets are effective tools for fat loss, increasing our energy expenditure and exposing us to a large number of movements.

Exercise	Sets	Reps	Rest	Tempo
A1. Lunge A2. DB Press A3. KB Deadlift A4. Lat Pulldown	3	10-12R	60s	3010
B1. Goblet Squat B2. DB Row B3. Hip Thrust B4. DB Shoulder Press	3	10-12R	60s	3010

Figure 7.6

CIRCUITS

This refers to any combination of exercises greater than four consecutive movements. Circuits are fun, and they are commonly used for group classes to create an engaging, challenging environment. It's mentally stimulating to engage in such a barrage of different exercises. We can use this for overload techniques, such as completing as many rounds or reps as possible within a given timeframe before moving on to the next movement. Circuits are ideal end points for people wanting to improve their body composition through losing fat mass and their anaerobic and aerobic capacity.

Exercise	Sets	Reps	Rest	Tempo
A1. Goblet Squat A2. DB Press A3. KB Deadlift A4. Lat Pulldown A5. Core A6. Calf Riase	3	10-12R	60s	3010

Figure 7.7

ANTAGONIST SETS

An antagonist set is a superset that is focused on opposing muscles. Opposing muscles exist and work in synergy throughout our body to achieve movement. One muscle will contract, and the opposing relaxes to allow our bone orientation to shift, thus creating a change in motion.

When writing a programme focusing on antagonist muscles, an easy way to think about this is training our chest and back together. We might perform one set of push-ups (pushing motion), followed by a set of rows (pulling motion); this, together, creates an antagonist set.

The benefit of this style of training is that it allows us to maintain a relatively high intensity with maximum efficiency. As opposed to straight sets that we previously mentioned, where I perform a set, rest for a minute or two, then repeat, I can now perform my chest and back movement and then rest, for say one minute instead two. My opposing muscle is effectively resting while the agonist is working, which allows for a time-efficient structure.

Exercise	Sets	Reps	Rest	Tempo
A1. Leg Extension A2. Leg Curl	3	10-12R	60s	3010
B1. DB Chest Press B2. DB Bent over row	3	10-12R	60s	3010

Figure 7.8

AGONIST SETS

An agonist set is more of a technique or method to elicit greater progressive overload. I will often use this with an intermediate or advanced trainee.

While the antagonist method pairs two OPPOSING muscles together, an agonist pairs two of the SAME muscles together.

The result? A nasty combination that will leave you desperate to take advantage of every second of your rest period. For these types of sets, we will typically require an extended rest period. I would advise not to use this in a strength-based programme as the fatigue it creates will lead to a reduced output in your strength.

So, why would we use this?

We can maximise our volume in a short amount of time: four sets effectively become eight sets for that muscle group in the workout. Generally, due to the accumulation of peripheral fatigue, we will require at least 90 seconds up to three or four minutes for rest periods to ensure we recover and can maintain a decent intensity in our proceeding sets and exercises.

Exercise	Sets	Reps	Rest	Tempo
A1. Goblet Squats A2. Leg Extension	3	10-12R	120s	3010
B1. Bench Press B2. Push Ups	3	10-12R	120s	3010

Figure 7.9

ADVANCED TECHNIQUES

I want to preface this section with the notion that these techniques are essentially not required for people new to training e.g. any novice trainees.

These techniques should be utilised by those doing intermediate to advanced training. Why? Well, I'm a great believer that we should train smarter not harder, for one. We know through much research that novices can get away with a lot less stimulus than an advanced trainer. With so much going on, such as exposure to different movements, being in a new environment, the physical and psychological demands, why bother adding an unnecessarily difficult training method when you can get away with some simple straight or super sets?

When formatting these advanced techniques, pay attention to the variables that are manipulated: the sets, reps, rest, tempo, format, exercise selection and positioning of our body will all play a part in getting the result we desire.

DROP SETS

The drop set is first on our list of advanced overloading techniques. A drop set refers to completing your normal set of straight sets, super sets, whatever style you choose, followed by a 10-30% drop in the weight of the load.

We can do this once or repeated times depending on what we want and how advanced we are. This may look like completing a set of squats at 100kg. Immediately afterwards, we reduce the weight to somewhere between 70kg and 90kg and go again, either for a predetermined set of reps or until we can do no more. By doing this, we activate our muscle fibres as much as possible under tension, giving us a better chance of gaining muscle hypertrophy, strength and eliciting peripheral nervous system fatigue.

This type of programming will be useful for those who wish to elicit hypertrophy and are short on time but wish to maintain volume and relative intensity.

Exercise	Sets	Reps	Rest	Tempo
1.Bench Press	3	10-12R w/ 2 x Drop Sets after each set	120s	3010
2. Deadlift	3	10-12R w/ 2 x Drop Sets after each set	120s	3010

Figure 7.10

Reverse sequencing

Now, I know I'm contradicting myself here, but reverse sequencing is where I sometimes break my rule of not exposing novices to advanced techniques. This might work well for some who are transitioning to intermediate training. Reverse sequencing is largely about how we format an exercise regime. It was mentioned earlier that what we train first, we train best. In a normal programme, we typically start with our large compound movements, the patterns we want to master. With reverse sequencing, this is not the case. Instead, we start with the smaller muscles we may often neglect, our accessories, such as our wrist flexors and extensors, our calves and so on. We then move into progressively larger and more complex movement types.

Let's use the example of a leg session. For this, I would typically programme a number of sets of calf exercises at the start of the workout, followed by open-chain exercises such as leg extensions and leg curls. Then we may look to programme more closed-chain movements, working up to our big compound movements of squatting, deadlifting, hip thrusting, etc.

This technique enables us to specialise within specific movements: we can practise our technique under fatigue, pre-exhaust certain muscles so we have no choice but to target other muscles that may be neglected. This is a way of creating a new stimulus if our training adaptations have plateaued. The downside, as you can guess, is that we will suffer in our movements later when we are fatigued. This has both pros and cons. Pros include targeting a specific muscle we want trained, as well as being able to reduce the load required to receive adaptation. The cons include minimising our ability to exert force, which has a negative result on people looking to gain strength. There is a trade-off with everything we do, after all.

This trade-off is one of the key reasons why I would potentially give this to a novice, as working on smaller areas will ensure that when we get to our larger movements, we physically cannot lift too much weight due to our peripheral fatigue. Now we can expose a novice to a multi-joint and muscle-recruiting exercise, such as a squat or deadlift, and receive adaptation under minimal load while also ensuring they develop their technique while fatigued. Win, win in my eyes.

Exercise	Sets	Reps	Rest	Tempo
A1. DB Hamer Curl A2. DB Tricep Extension	4	20R	60s	3010
B1. Push Ups B2. Inverted BB Rows (UH Grip)	4	10-12R	60s	3010
C1. DB Shoulder Press C2. Lat Pulldown (OH Grip)	3	10-12R	90s	3010
D1. Bench Press D2. Bent Over BB Rows	3	8-10R	120s	3010

Figure 7.11

REP MODIFICATIONS

Typically, a repetition involves moving a weight through its full range of motion, contracting and lengthening our muscle. With rep modification, we play around with these mechanics to create a new stimulus for our musculature. We can perform one and a quarter reps. If we were squatting, this means we would squat down as low as we can, come up partially (a quarter), and go back down to the bottom before standing up to complete one repetition. You can imagine this will affect a muscle by increasing its time under tension and eliciting metabolic stress, two key variables in promoting muscle hypertrophy. As a rule of thumb, due to their nature, these rep modifications are best suited for closed-chain exercises, meaning machines or positions where our legs and hands are fixed in position. These allow us to decrease the potential injury risk while creating the stimulus we require for our repetition modifications.

Exercise	Sets	Reps	Rest	Tempo
A1. Goblet Squats (1 & 1/4) A2. DB Press (1 & 1/4)	4	8-10R	90s	3010
B1. DB RDLs (1 & 1/4) B2. Lat Pulldown (1 & 1/4)	4	8-10R	90s	3010
C1. DB Shoulder Press C2. Lat Pulldown (OH Grip)	3	10-12R	90s	3010

Figure 7.12

ACCENTUATED REPS

Not all contractions are created equally. Just like with our energy systems, there's a sliding scale, with certain types of contractions favouring a higher output of force. Within each muscle contraction exists three possibilities:

1. The muscle shortens.

2. The muscle lengthens.

3. The muscle stays the same length.

Each type of contraction has a specific name: shortening is referred to as concentric; lengthening is referred to as eccentric; while our muscle staying the same length is called an isometric contraction. Eccentric, when our muscles lengthen, is the strongest, about 20% stronger than concentric. We can use this to our advantage with accentuated repetitions.

You can now use this information to alter how you overload on specific exercises.

Let's run through an example of accentuated reps for leg presses. Suppose that 100kg is a comfortable weight for you to lift with both legs but a struggle with one. The accentuated rep would involve using one leg to lower the weight down (eccentric contraction), then placing our second foot on the leg press platform and pushing it back up (concentric contraction). This is known as a supramaximal effort for the single limb, as it is exceeding its concentric ability.

We can accentuate the time as well by performing two-legged leg presses with excessively long eccentric portions, say 10 seconds of lowering the weight down before pressing the weight back up. **A simple way to think about this method is two up, one down.**

REST-PAUSE

The rest-pause method allows us to work in a high-intensity environment through the manipulation of our rest period. Typically, when using a rest-pause method, we will allocate an arbitrary number of repetitions for the set. For the sake of this example, let's say 40 reps. I will choose a weight that I can perform for roughly 10 repetitions (we are looking at around 70% to 80% of your maximum ability to lift). We perform our 10 reps and then rest for about 20 seconds. This is a very short time in the scheme of the set, with the aim of creating a form of metabolic stress and tension on the working muscles. We then proceed to perform as many reps as we can, and each time we need to stop we get a 20-second rest. This may get to a depressingly low number, even just one, before we require a rest – if we allocate the correct load. Generally, I would use this method for movements with low mechanical techniques to mitigate the risk of injury. An example for legs would be leg extension, while for the upper body it may involve performing lat pulldowns.

Exercise	Sets	Reps	Rest	Tempo
A1. DB Press	3	40R	10s rest between pauses, 2 minutes after completion	3010
B1. Leg Extension	3	40R	10s rest between pauses, 2 minutes after completion	3010
C1. DB Rows C2. Leg Curls	3	10-12R	60s	3010

Figure 7.13

STRENGTH-LOADING PROTOCOLS

Protocols change over time. For example, the research used to state that the 8-12 repetition range was the be-all and end-all for hypertrophy or muscle growth. This has since gone out the window, so to speak, with research showing we can stimulate hypertrophy within a range of 6-100 reps and onwards. This is not the case for strength, the repetition range for which has remained largely unchanged. With our strengthening protocols, we want to keep the repetitions to a minimum to maintain a high intensity. The rep range for this protocol is generally under five or less. This allows us to work with high intensity; the higher the intensity, the more muscle we must recruit to accomplish the task.

The protocols for developing strength are not subject to these ranges only; it is definitely possible to still gain strength using the 8-12 range. Our nervous system becomes more efficient, we can recruit an increased number of motor units (contractile units of muscle) and complete our jobs more effectively. We also know that there exists a threshold for adaptation. For lighter protocols, like 6-100 repetitions, this is really only effective in the last few repetitions. For example, if I was using 5kg and performing bicep curls, I may be able to do this for 60 reps before I failed. Now, if I stopped at 40 reps on a set, I will not be providing sufficient overload stimulus to incur adaptation to the area. That is due to the amount of muscle activation I am eliciting.

As we fatigue, we need to recruit more motor units to complete the task. At 40 reps, let's say 70% of the motor units in my muscles are recruited; at 60 reps this may stimulate 100% of my motor units. This is called Henneman's size principle, which states "that as more force is required, motor units will be recruited in a precise order according to the magnitude of force output".

Think of this principle like boiling water in a kettle. As we first turn on the kettle, the water is cold (low motor unit recruitment); as we wait and more heat (stimulus) is applied to the kettle, the water starts to increase its temperature (time under tension). After sufficient time with the water heating, a chemical reaction occurs leading to the water boiling. Our muscle is similar: at the beginning we only use so much; but as time goes on that we are working the muscle, we must activate it more to continue performing the task. As we approach the climax of our set, we activate our muscle completely, leaving us to reap the rewards of providing enough stimulus for change.

Now, if we start off with 5kg and performed five reps, a minimal amount of our muscle would be recruited in this range, relatively speaking. If instead, we used 30kg, the demand for force output is significantly increased from the get-go. This would require the stimulation of a far greater number of motor units to achieve the task of lifting the weight, making it more effective for strength adaptations.

To recap – if you want to get strong, it is more efficient to lift heavy objects for a few reps.

Keep this in mind when you are writing a programme for a specific component such as strength; you might wish to alter the format of your programme to place your strength-based exercises at the start (we know what we do first, we do best), keeping it under around five repetitions to give us an ideal environment for gains. We also know that increased rest is required for repeated intensity efforts, so for our strength protocols we will require longer rest periods (two to three minutes at least). The way we format an exercise can vary greatly, as you should now be becoming aware.

WAVE LOADING

With this technique, we perform a descending or ascending order of repetitions, like a pyramid. This, in my experience, is a brilliant way of developing strength while adding some variety.

To perform this method, we may start at five reps, then perform three reps, followed by just one rep. Throughout this, we will progressively change the weight, and the overall intensity will increase as volume or reps decrease. I will generally programme wave loading in a 7-5-3R format or 6-4-2R or 5-3-1R.

We perform six sets, working through 5-3-1R scheme for our first three, then we return back to five reps in the fourth, three reps in the fifth and one rep in the sixth set. Only on these occasions, with more weight than the first time we did it.

HERE'S AN EXAMPLE:

Set 1 - 5R @ - 80% 1 Rep Max (RM)

Rest

Set 2 - 3R @ - 85% 1RM

Rest

Set 3 - 1R @ 90% 1RM

Rest

Set 4 - 5R @ 82.5% 1RM

Rest

Set 5 – 3R @ 87.5% 1RM

Rest

Set 6 – 1R @92.5% 1RM

As you can see, we have progressively increased the percentage of our 1 rep maximum. This is another physiological trick that we can use. The wave-like nature of this rep scheme encourages us to stimulate high-threshold motor units to elicit greater force output. Then, when we increase the repetitions again, we can lift the loads more comfortably in our fourth set than we could in our first set through the priming effect of the previous exposures.

It's worth mentioning that, in my opinion, outside of specific sports such as powerlifting I don't see the need to test or work towards a one-repetition maximum. For me, the cons, such as heightening the risk of injury and taxing the central nervous system, outweigh the pros. The lowest I typically take someone is three repetitions for their maximum, most commonly seen in a

7-5-3 wave-loading format. This still has good carry-over to your potential maximum without ego training.

Exercise	Sets	Reps	Rest	Tempo
A1. BB Shoulder Press	6	7-5-3R	120-180s	3010
B1. BB Deadlift	6	7-5-3R	120-180s	3010
C1. DB Shoulder Press C2. KB Swings	4	10-12R	60s	3010

Figure 7.14

CLUSTER SETS

Cluster sets are another great training method that allows us to perform exercise with a high relative load while significantly reducing the potential for injury. How? This lies in the way we perform our reps and alter our rest periods.

In the cluster set, we 'cluster' or condense our set into small efforts or repetitions. A normal strength exercise may see you perform six consecutive repetitions; in the cluster, we still perform six repetitions but we space this out.

We may perform two repetitions then rest for a small amount of time, then another two, then rest, then another two to complete our first set of six repetitions. This mitigates the injury risk as our form can remain intact rather than grinding out the fifth and sixth repetitions; we now get to reset and compose ourselves before we lift the weight again.

The downside is that it's difficult to rely on our stretch-short-ening reflex, aka momentum or touch-and-go lifting due to the stop-start nature of the method. For example, in the deadlift, we pause after the second rep, take a 30-second rest and then re-engage for the lift. Pulling the bar from the floor initially is where many people struggle with this movement, so performing six consecutive repetitions usually allows people to make the movement more easily by relying on our elastic muscle proper-ties. This is known as the recoiling effect, which helps us bounce back up into the next rep. By having a pause, momentum is taken away and we must essentially generate more force to lift the weight, leading to higher fatigue overall. Nonetheless, I view the cluster set as a very powerful method of eliciting strength while keeping the fatigue minimal and therefore reducing the injury risk to the individual.

Exercise	Sets	Reps	Rest	Tempo
A1. BB Shoulder Press	6	2-2-2R	30s between each 2R then 2 minutes after 6R	3010
B1. BB Deadlift	6	2-2-2R	30s between each 2R then 2 minutes after 6R	3010
C1. DB Shoulder Press C2. KB Swings	3	10-12R	60s	3010

Figure 7.15

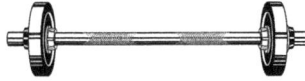

OVERVIEW

The methods explained in this chapter are just a few ways we can manipulate variables to achieve an outcome. What I want you to take away from this chapter in particular is the wide choice available to us when we understand the basic principles of training. Think back to the concepts of a good programme. Whether it's for a client or yourself, it is good practice to create sustainable and effective outcome-based programmes. If you start your first training programme with agonist, drop sets and use all these crazy methods, chances are you will hate yourself and me for giving you the idea, leading to low adherence, failure to reach your goals and death.

Ok, maybe not actual death, but the death of your goal at least, whatever that may be. Be patient when starting your journey. No one starts off a video game with the ability to beat the boss at the end of the game, you must earn the right to fight them through the blood, sweat and tears you will shed and the knowledge you gain throughout your journey.

Now, when it comes to your health there is no big bad boss, and hopefully, you will only shed sweat and not blood and tears, but you get the idea. Don't try and conquer health and fitness in week one; view it as a marathon, not a sprint. There is a certain rite of passage that must be navigated through our programming. We must lay the foundation for more advanced movements and techniques with our initial programmes. There should be a sequential flow in what we expose ourselves and/or our clients to. This will be covered in depth through our periodisation chapter.

8

Systems, Systems, Systems

"They always say time changes things, but you actually have to change them yourself." -Andy Warhol

T his chapter is all about periodisation, which refers to the planning, design and execution of our programmes and training to elicit progression and specific peaking or maximal output in our chosen area.[32] A goal can and should be broken up into achievable long- and short-term steps, more on this in Chapter 12. That is, in essence, periodising.

We must align our programmes or training to match the required outcomes, at the specific time we need them. What use is attaining the strength or athletic ability to perform at our peak ability during the off-season when it's required the least? Or fulfilling our KPI quota at work three months after it is due.

How effective is our programme if we achieve our goal too late?

Knowing when and how to ramp up our programming or actionable steps to achieve a goal is just as important as the goals themselves. This is the biggest role we have to play. We must orchestrate an intelligent programme to enable our dreams to come true in a timely and appropriate manner.

Periodising involves three key variables: the macrocycles, the mesocycles and the microcycles. Periodisation does not just have to apply merely to training or exercise. Keep an open mind and you can apply this knowledge to multiple facets of your life to get the outcome you desire.

MACROCYCLE

Think of this as the big picture. It is the foundation upon which you can build, the long-term goal if you will. A simple example is if we were an athlete working towards the Olympics, which happens every four years (unless COVID-19 throws it out the window). That period is our large macrocycle. We know we need to perform at our peak in four years' time, and at certain events along the way if we are to even qualify.

MESOCYCLE

The mesocycle is the specific phase within our macrocycle training programme. I dare say this is the most important step. We have set ourselves a macrocycle, but if we fail to action it within specific phases (mesocycles) we will have little success in reaching our goal. Typically, a mesocycle will be three to four weeks in length.

Let's start in January. We have a goal of reaching peak performance in the sport of weightlifting by November (this is our macrocycle). To do this, we must break our goal into mesocycles – phases that allow us to target certain areas. For this person starting in January, we could break them into 12 mesocycles (one-month blocks), which also allows for a period of recovery. This plan can be written a number of different ways based on the desired outcome. For example, you might have to 'perform at your best in trials halfway through the year to qualify for the competition in November. This would require you to ramp up your training before downregulating it for recovery and then re-ramping as you approach the big event.

Here is an example of 12 mesocycles.

Phase 1 – January to March: focusing on general preparation for the task at hand. Within these mesocycles will exist four-week programmes, increasing in technicality as we move into more specific areas of training in a later phase.

In your everyday life you could use this period to plan and figure out what you require to reach your goal, say x number of sales so you get a bonus. This is where you may scope out your competition, look at potential buyers and thoroughly research the product you are selling.

Phase 2 – April to June: we may start to look at accruing volume for our weightlifting competition through an accumulation phase. This basically means we have higher levels of volume and frequency. This may involve a linear progression of our repetition schemes, starting at higher ranges such as three sets of 12-15 repetitions, before moving to four sets of 8-12 repetitions in the second mesocycle of this phase and finishing with five or six sets of 4-6 repetitions.

In the everyday life example, you start to accumulate sales. You call, email, and door knock, getting progressively more aggressive in your sales tactics as the month's progress. You may look to expand your territory.

Phase 3 – July to September: our pre-competition phase. This is when we want to dial down on the technical components, balance out our intensity with our recovery and maintain our abilities.

You are approaching your sales target, but you face competition. Now you must hone your skills of persuasion and persistence to keep your competitors at bay.

Phase 4 – October to December: it's go time. Here, we can enter a specialisation phase, again made up of three mesocycles. In October we will intensify the programme, in November we will peak and taper our programme, in December we will recover. Each mesocycle will use different constraints around the format – sets, repetitions, recovery and order of our programme – to elicit the best possible outcome within our designated time.

Your sales peak until you reach your target. You get ready for a presentation to your boss on the deadline date. You demonstrate what you have achieved to your boss, earning that bonus. You now realise how exhausted you have been due to all the hard work, so it's time for a much-needed holiday with your family!

MICROCYCLE

The microcycle is the daily or weekly actions required to make up the mesocycles and macrocycles. Much like with goal setting, here lies the actionable steps, the small events we participate in regularly that add up to our large end goal. The microcycle is the shortest type of training cycle, and here we use block programming. We may allocate specific days for training or resting. Monday may be a push day, Tuesday may be a pull day, Wednesday may be rest, Thursday may be our cardio day and so on until we make up a week's worth of programming.

You can get creative with the variables here. They can be manipulated in countless ways to make up the larger mesocycles and macrocycles. This is where we need to match the training with the lifestyle of the individual. If we set the task of training seven days per week but only have time for four days, we will fail.

Time to put this together!

Cycle	Phase 1 Jan - Mar		Phase 2 Apr - June		Phase 3 July - Sept		Phase 4 Oct - Dec	
Macro	Preparation Phase (0-6 Months)				Competition Phase (7-12 Months)			
Meso	General Preparation		Accumulation		Specific Phase and Maintenance		Peak and Tapering	
Micro								

Figure 8.1

The macrocycle is based on our yearly goal, in this instance split into two distinct phases – the preparation phase and the competition phase. The mesocycle is based on 12 cycles (a month each). These are split into further subgroups – general preparation, accumulation, specific preparation and maintenance and peaking and tapering. Lastly, the microcycles are based on one-week blocks. Combined, these form a yearly training plan.

Now, I've mentioned a couple of terms that you may not be aware of – peaking and tapering. Let me elaborate.

Peaking

This allows us to achieve our peak performance. It is what all our periodising is moving towards, the end goal of being our best at a certain point in time. In order to peak, our training programme needs to account for variables of volume, frequency, intensity and recovery if we are to get the best out of ourselves. Peaking goes hand in hand with tapering.

Tapering

Tapering is an important part of a periodisation plan. To employ this technique, we must respect the principle of recovery and rest directly before the peak performance is required. To taper, we must deliberately reduce the intensity and/or volume to minimise any cumulative fatigue that may have arisen since the start of our training or life endeavours. Tapering works on more than just the physical; it has been shown to positively improve mood, reduce the sense of fatigue and act as a reset for the individual to engage in their activity again with significantly more ease. Basically, you can't just keep taking on work tasks forever without burning out. Something must give. To be at your best, you need phases of highs and lows. This is where tapering comes in; it allows you to exert a level of control in when to be at your best.

We need to be careful here – remember the principle of reversibility? If we spend too long resting, we risk a decrease in our performance. Tapering must be carefully executed to ensure that all our efforts lead us to perform at our peak. Common tapering recommendations involve reducing training times between eight and 14 days before the peak is required, while maintaining a decent intensity or volume to avoid detraining. This is a rest, but not a vacation; the person is still required to work throughout this period, just at a reduced rate e.g., 50%-60% of their usual amount.

TEST, THEN RETEST

We now have a sound understanding of the variables that can go into planning and executing our training programme. The question remains, how do we know if we are being effective? We test! Periodic testing can help determine if we need to alter our path, our plan towards excellence, or if we can stay as we are. An example of what might cause us to veer off the path would be holidays, key life events or sometimes injury.

It is worth having a theoretical toolbox of techniques you can employ; the list below will give a number of ideas I've found useful, but keep in mind not all people are created equally so I will not be giving you a specific technique. Feel free to venture outside of these to find your own.

Journaling, rating of perceived exertion (RPE) scales, psychology questionnaires and performance outcomes are some of my favourite tools for assessing the effectiveness of a periodised programme.

- Journaling may involve writing down and tracking a series of metrics, rating them from one to 10, for example, with one pitting you as a horrendous sad sack and 10 being on top of the world. The metrics you track and measure can range from your mood, energy levels, sleep quality and quantity, and your perceived level of effort with tasks. I find this is a useful technique over longer periods. When we are reaching low numbers for a concerning amount of time (let's say two weeks) then it's time to assess what is going on, what we can change and how we can prevent overtraining.

Steve Jobs had a saying: "I have looked in the mirror every morning and asked myself: 'If today were the last day of my life, would I want to do what I am about to do today?' and whenever the answer has been 'No' for too many days in a row, I know I need to change something."

- RPE scales are always useful in the context of performance. Determining the rate of perceived exertion for an activity can go a long way in helping to modify a programme. The RPE scales rating system is basically inverse to that of journaling: 10 is difficult, and you can't do this for very long at high volumes or you might implode; whereas one on the scale is a walk in the park, you could do this till the cows come home, so to speak. With such little effort, you risk not achieving any significant adaptation to your training and will potentially fail to reach your goal.

- Psychology questionnaires can be useful in determining fatigue levels and RPE; it's another form of journaling. There are a number of valid and reliable questionnaires out there, dependent on what you are trying to achieve. A quick Google search using the relevant term, such as readiness questionnaire or anxiety questionnaire, can help you find the right one.

- Does it feel like you're suddenly back in the cognitive stage of your skill? Are you missing sessions or having difficulty with movements you once completed effortlessly? This can be a key factor in determining how ready you are for performance (readiness). How you respond to a training stimulus and the rate of decline can determine how aggressive you should be with your approach to changing your programme or other factors of your life that may be contributing to a drop in performance.

OVERREACHING

Overreaching can be both beneficial and determinantal to our performance. This generally occurs through a build-up of fatigue from both training and non-training stimuli. Functional overreaching (the beneficial kind) can enable us to develop physiological adaptations to compensate for the stress we have undergone days or weeks prior. Let's use the example of delayed onset muscle soreness (DOMS). We're in the gym to train a specific set of muscles, and in the following 24 to 72 hours we experience a decrease in our performance as our body recovers. We're sore and the stress has taken hold of us. Our body is striving to adapt, so next time we overcome this, low and behold we get physiological adaptations. Now, DOMS isn't actually a good measure of progress – you don't need to be sore to adapt (this process is much more complex than the above example, but you get the point). Non-functional overreaching, as defined by Meeusen and colleagues, is classified as applying a stimulus for a long period of time, exceeding the person's ability to recover and resulting in a stagnation or decrease in performance output.[33] This brings us to overtraining.

OVERTRAINING

The dreaded overtraining. This affects our ability to perform and is something we wish to avoid at all costs. It's the reason we employ our toolbox of tracking metrics. Overtraining can lead to both physical and psychological alterations within the body. It can disturb our nervous system, disrupt its normal function, affect our ability to recruit muscles, increase our heart rate and blood pressure at rest and compromise our immune function. This is just to name a few negative associations with overtraining. I think you get the point. Avoid this at all costs.

We should monitor our metrics and prevent extended over-reaching so it does not lead to overtraining. We can manipulate volume, intensity, fatigue, exercise selection, stressors, format-ting and other variables to mitigate the effects of overtraining.

ENVIRONMENT

For the general population, this variable will be less important; for athletes or people working towards a goal that may encounter them having to adapt to perform in different humidity and temperatures, the environment will be much more important. We need time to adapt to our surroundings, much like we need time to adapt to our training. Seasonal sports such as soccer and netball will have their pre-season training basically in the opposite climate to when they compete e.g., summer vs. winter. In our working life, acclimatising to the environment may be viewed through the lens of the busy season (tax time) vs. the holiday season. We must account for this through our programmes.

The technicality and level of periodisation will depend on your ability to understand and organise the large number of components we have discussed so far, whether it's a programme for training, sports, work or life in general.

To recap, periodising is essential in all facets of our life: sport, career, recreation, you name it. Our long-term goal (macrocycle) can be broken down into medium goals, or monthly targets (mesocycle) and even small goals, or daily habits (microcycle). These are all important in the journey to achieving our peak performance when the time comes.

We can monitor the effectiveness of our programmes through metrics of difficulty, fatigue, stress and recovery. Tracking these metrics will allow us to view data over time so we can recalibrate as needed, giving us the ideal environment to overreach rather than overtrain.

We can't go at something 100% all the time. Be smart and plan for success. Look at when you need to be your best, and plan regular intervals of rest and recovery, known as tapering, so we can let our bodies recover both physically and psychologically. This will allow us to reach our peak. To truly peak, we need to account for not just the physical but also the psychological. In the next chapter, we will delve into the psychology of mindset.

9

Be Plastic

"Every thought we think is creating our future."
-Louise Hay

O ur mind is powerful. Have you ever considered the way our mind (psychology) can affect us physically?

Psychology is inseparable from any form of physical activity. The motivations behind why we embark on certain goals, how we perceive difficulty, how are energy levels are, how we manage and perceive stress and how we regularly behave come from our mind.

If you are planning on engaging in an exercise programme with the intention of adopting a healthier behaviour, first seek to understand your mindset.

Understanding one's psychology is a form of intelligence, coined emotional intelligence. The definition of emotional intelligence is "the ability to understand, use, and manage your own emotions in positive ways to relieve stress, communicate effectively, empathize with others, overcome challenges and defuse conflict". Why am I talking about emotions and mindset in the same paragraph? you ask.

Humans are more than just physical. We are comprised of emotions, hormones, experiences, environments and thoughts as well as our bodies themselves. So far within this book, we have largely focused on the physical. This is easy for most people to grasp: we can see our bodies, we can touch them, it's a tangible concept.

The mind is different. We can't see our mind, we can't touch our mind, instead it is just there. In my experience, this is a much more difficult concept for people to grasp. We know our minds exist, but we may underestimate the power they have, the ability to change us physiologically for better or worse.

So, ask yourself what makes you, you?

What experiences, beliefs, attitudes, systems and people have you been exposed to that have shaped the way your mind works?

The mind is a muscle, and, like any muscle, in order for it to grow, we must provide it with sufficient stimulus to encourage adaptation and change. This can be in the form of experiences, beliefs, attitudes, systems and people we encounter throughout various stages of our lives. The mind follows the same principles that we apply to muscles: progressive overload, adaptation, specificity, reversibility and recovery.

To explain how this works with progressive overload and adaptation, let's use an example of studying for a test. We can approach this in two simple ways.

Option one: we study over a period of weeks, gradually building on our previous foundation of knowledge and layering the new information on top to allow us to learn and understand the content in broader and more complex scenarios.

Option two: we put off all study until the night before. Many of us will be familiar with this style, known as cramming.

We try and condense months' worth of content into one night and retain it all.

Generally, option two is much less effective compared to option one. If we compare this to training, do you expect to receive all of the muscle adaptation you possibly can by engaging in one workout? Well, maybe some people new to exercise will have that belief but they would be very misguided. We need progressive, repeated exposure followed by recovery over a sustained period of time to create our desired level of change, and the mind is no different. If it is to learn, grow and develop into a stronger, more resilient tool, it too needs to be progressively overloaded with stimulus.

This stimulus can be positive, such as learning new skills; creating, reflecting, reading and using the power of our mind to actively work through solutions to whatever problems we may face. It can also be negative, where we progressively overload our minds by scrolling through endless social media content i.e., Facebook and Instagram, engaging in poor conversations or watching hours of TV..

Feel free to progressively overload your minds with information about your favourite topics. In my case, that's the art and science of the physiology behind why our bodies function the way they do. My stimulus is learning the intricacies of the body as a whole, ranging from the physiological underpinnings that keep you alive to the way you talk and hold yourself.

Don't spread yourself too thin when it comes to stimulating your mind, as this can have negative consequences. I think you should follow your passion. Have you ever intended to study for a test only to find yourself in a deep, dark hole watching countless YouTube videos that have no relation to your life? This is an example of being unfocused with our attention, delving into less-than-ideal circumstances for mind stimulation.

How many people do you know that complain about their jobs, their relationships, and their lives? I bet there are even some of you reading this agreeing that you hate where you are right now. Alan Watts, the great, late philosopher, gave me some perspective on this matter of the mind when he asked: "What would you be doing with your life if money were no object?" I pondered this, and I encourage you to do the same. Really dedicate the time and attention this deserves, as it will enable you to determine your path. Set aside distractions, switch off social media and get in touch with yourself. Look at who you are now, what dreams you had as a child and where you want to be five, 10 even 20 years from now. What steps must you take to remember who you are?

In some instances, this is where you will be required to apply the principle of reversibility. Contrary to our muscular or physical systems, this principle can often be an invaluable tool for our minds. Before you call me crazy, let me explain. The principle of reversibility states that we lose any gains once we stop engaging with a certain activity. This, like many of the concepts we have covered, can be beneficial or determinantal to us. Try and view reversibility as a positive: how many times in our lives have we been exposed to poor influences – environments, thoughts, feelings, people and decisions? We may have engaged with a particularly destructive behaviour such as smoking cigarettes, maybe you still do. This is where we can use the principle of reversibility to our advantage within our minds. Discover your negative behaviours, and then you can find a way to reverse them. This could be how you speak to yourself, the beliefs you have been taught but no longer agree with or the fears and vulnerabilities that have developed throughout your life. All can be undone. Our minds are versatile; we can unwire and rewire our brains to learn and unlearn a large majority of what we know, think and feel.

Do you allow your mind to recover? Have you ever longed for bed after an extremely long day at work? Have you ever craved a vacation or just felt lethargic for no apparent reason? Your mind, like your muscles, requires recovery. This may be in the form of a holiday, meditation or frequent practices of mindfulness. The mind can impact us physically if it's drained; it can cause us to be fatigued, impacting our mood and our nervous system.

Our mind is the fuel for our vehicle. Your hobbies in life could be considered your recovery system. What do you enjoy doing? This falls in line with our previous paragraph regarding specificity: there exists specific activities in each of our lives that can recharge or drain us. Find the balance between these, both are necessary.

I could write another book rather than just a chapter on the mind. It is barely understood, yet what we do know is incredible. To exhibit the power of our minds, let's look at a number of experiments carried out throughout the years.

Placebo, nocebo

The placebo effect is a phenomenon commonly explored within clinical research trials which demonstrates the power of the mind over matter. An example you may have heard of is the sugar pill, often used in the research phase of developing a new pharmaceutical drug. Participants will be divided into two groups, a control group that takes the placebo (sugar pill) and another that takes the drug they are looking to test.

The placebo is literally just sugar, nothing fancy about it whatsoever. The trick lies in what the subjects are told. They are made to think this sugar pill is the actual drug, capable of potential benefits., This could be anything from a reduction in blood pressure to improved strength, speed and endurance. Sounds too good to be true, doesn't it?

This is a well-researched concept, and everything points to the mind as the culprit behind why a placebo can work. The plain and simple explanation is that what the mind believes capable, becomes capable.

Placebos affect people differently. Why? you ask. Well, this is largely attributed to the weight of belief the subject places in the object. Those susceptible to a placebo often light up an area of their brain's basal ganglia known as the nucleus accumbens. The role of this area is to tie in motivation with action, basically a reward centre.

The belief of the practitioner can also have an impact – their conviction and communication style e.g., a doctor administering the drugs versus someone less qualified.

Let's explore the devilish sibling of the placebo, the dreaded nocebo effect. I feel like a broken record writing this, but it's worth noting again that there exists a continuum between positive and negative benefits. Anything seemingly positive can become negative, with the placebo being no exception. This brings us to the nocebo effect, where people are basically told the opposite: that this pill, activity, action, will harm them, cause negative effects. What's the result? Well, as you have probably guessed, they start to feel those negative effects. There is even research to suggest that someone simply not being aware of the side effects of a medication can change the influence it has on them. So, feelings of nausea, for example, could be a by-product of you thinking you will get nausea from taking a medication, all because you read that this is a possible side effect. Crazy, huh! [34]

What's even more fascinating is that the nocebo can even overpower common medications that have been shown to work! Researchers have identified people with pain, given them a documented pain-relieving drug and seen improvements as expected. These subjects were later told that their pain would come back if they stopped taking this genuine drug. The interesting finding of this study was that the subjects stopped feeling the benefits immediately, even while they were still consuming the product.

Thus, cancelling out any benefits the drug once had for them due to their new belief.[35]

Now that we have discussed the potential positive and negative effects of the placebo and nocebo phenomena, is it too far of a stretch to take this a step further and apply this to what we tell ourselves, the ideas we entertain, our thoughts, beliefs and behaviours?

If a sugar pill can cause physical symptoms because our mind believes it to be a real drug, then I'd suggest we can take that step.

THE STANFORD PRISON EXPERIMENT

This experiment is famous for being one of the most profound psychological studies in history. It studied the psychology of people when placed in a different environment. Subjects were randomly split into two groups, the prisoners and the guards, roles which they had to fulfill for the length of the study, 24 hours a day. All had a healthy medical history, no known psychological issues, and no criminal charges against them.[36]

Despite its worldwide fame, this study was never even completed. Why? Because of the huge impact it was having on the subjects' behaviour. The guards had become violent, abusive and aggressive towards the inmates. The inmates began to experience anxiety, stress and fear. Why did this occur? The participants were forced to believe in their mind that they held a specific role, and this affected them a significant portion morally and socially. On one side, the guards were given the moral high ground, to look over people who were to be considered inferior wrongdoers. On the other side, the inmates, people who in real life had no criminal record, were made to believe they were guilty, corrupt and somewhat deserving of this punishment. Their environment influenced their mindsets. The result? A fundamental behaviour change.

Now, let's apply this to you. Have you been brought up to believe you have a predetermined role? Do your parents, your friends or your family hold certain beliefs about you? They may have wanted a specific career path, a doctor or lawyer, for example. Due to the environment they have created, have you formed new characteristics to meet these expectations?

Japan and South Korea both have high rates of suicide and high rates of job satisfaction. A confounding situation? Absolutely, but situations like this are found throughout the world. This stimulates thoughts and questions within my own mind.

What environments, expectations and behaviours exist within our own society to cause such high instances of poor physical and mental health worldwide? Can this come down to our mindset? The belief that we can learn and unlearn what we have been taught? I believe this is a key factor in engaging in healthier behaviours throughout your life. The ability to be resilient, persevere and welcome the challenge at hand stem from your mindset.

So far, we have covered the power of our mind, and how it is an integral influence on our beliefs and behaviours.

Continue reading as we venture into the two predominant mindsets that we form – fixed and growth – that determine every decision and action we make.

MINDSET FORMATION

People will favour either a fixed or a growth mindset. You may have already heard of these concepts, and I guarantee that you have been in both at various stages throughout your life depending on the activity undertaken. These mindsets impact every situation in our lives because they determine the way we talk, think and feel.

Fixed mindset

Having a fixed mindset is like not being able to touch your toes. It's inflexible, rigid and unwavering. This mindset is one of limitation, boundaries and roadblocks. A person exhibiting this mindset may appear defensive, closed-minded and unwilling to accept any feedback or criticism. They will be reluctant to accept or acknowledge opinions different to their own. A fixed mindset keeps us within our comfort zone; it allows us to play it safe and avoid the uncomfortableness of reversing or undoing our belief systems and questioning ourselves. Fixed mindsets can present themselves in subtle and not-so-subtle ways. This may look like a professor who teaches in a way that has been proven ineffective because this is all they know. It is associated with phrases we say to explain away certain behaviour, such as "boys will be boys" or "a zebra never changes its stripes". These statements are absolutes, there's no potential for change.

Growth mindset

On the other hand, a growth mindset is like the ocean, in a constant state of flow. It can change, bend and break. Bruce Lee's quote, "Be like water", comes to mind. The ability to flow and crash, be strong and stern yet malleable. The ability to change shape as required. This is, in essence, a mind that greets opportunity. Someone with a growth mindset will be open, listen actively and demonstrate a willingness to alter their perspective when shown an alternative. These people embody phrases such as "if there's a will, there's a way" or "fall seven times, stand up eight". These phrases promote change, they relish a challenge and explore a vastness of scenarios to find the answer. These mindsets are shared by people of exploration, creation and ability. The growth mindset encourages adaptation, it encourages us to make mistakes and learn alternative solutions to problems. The growth mindset has led to technological, sporting and lifestyle advancements that have pushed the human race forward.

Let's put both of these mindsets into a scenario to highlight the contrast between them. We are at the local farmers' markets, and two farmers are selling their products – apples. Now, these two farmers have sold this type of apple their entire lives, but recently sales have dropped. Customers have been asking for a new type of apple. The first farmer, Frank, says he will never change the type of apples he sells; this is what the people have always liked and this is what they will get. It is all he knows, so why should Frank spend money and time learning about a new type of apple?

Gregory, the other farmer, listens to his customers and begins to stock a variety of apples. Frank's stall barely survives selling the same apple he always has, while Gregory's business flourishes and he receives more praise and profit than in all his previous years of selling apples.

Einstein said: "Insanity is repeating the same task over and over and expecting a different result." This quote comes to mind with Frank. He has a fixed mindset, decides not to change his view and is closed to the possibility of growing a variety of apples. Gregory's growth mindset means he views the art of growing apples as a constant endeavour of improvement. He embraces the challenge of learning new skills and information, which leads him to success.

What views, beliefs and absolutes do you hold? Write them down. You might write "I believe that the Earth is round". We know this to be true, but why? An activity I like to use is 'mind mapping', where I break down the events or experiences that have led to developing my beliefs. Akin to a family tree, we can trace back moments within our life that have led us down a path of adopting certain assumptions. I may now say that I believe that the Earth is round due to the scientific literature. This applies to your career paths, religion, outlook on life and basically every construct you think about. Take the time to discover where and why you are the way you are, then you will develop the power and ability to use your mind to your advantage. This will enable you to engage with a growth mindset. Being aware of your beliefs is the first step towards potentially altering them. Some of your beliefs will be positive, but some ways of thinking will result in us being destructive. Left unchecked, this can affect our lives in a variety of ways.

Find a quiet place when mind mapping. List down all the key parts of your life. For many of us this will be work/business, relationships, sport/leisure/recreation, and passion. As if going back in time on a family tree, look at influences for each of them – this may be certain beliefs, quotes or affirmations you commonly think of or say that have shaped your current lifestyle.

As your tree grows, you may find biased, outdated beliefs that can be updated. Look to grow the branches – what do you want to learn next to help you on your journey?

Taking time to assess your values and beliefs is an important step in understanding yourself. When you do, no one can take that away. If you've ever been bullied or, worse, you actually believed the bully, they hold the power over you because they in essence control who you are. They have told you who you are or aren't because you haven't taken the time to figure it out yourself. Self-knowledge can act as a shield against such attacks. This isn't to say words won't ever affect you again, rather it will help develop a raw power that enables you to be accountable and responsible for yourself. Knowing one's strengths and weaknesses is one of the most profound things we can teach ourselves.

Within a clinical context, I will often come across a variety of people with different attitudes and beliefs about why they have sought out my services. These people can be closed or open; they can have negative associations with my type of treatment, for example, people telling me that "they are too old for exercise" or "they walk at work so they don't need exercise" or "they have seen 10 other practitioners already". These people have developed a pattern of thinking, they are in a fixed mindset, and part of my job is firstly to show them another perspective or mindset. Then, I work with them to create healthy behaviours, educating them about the benefits of exercise and the like within this book, supplying the information they need to take control of their health.

If two people are unable to communicate and find common ground, then irrespective of the topic at hand a conversation will be of little use. To alter one's perspective – changing the mind from a fixed state to one of growth and sustenance – you must speak the same language. This doesn't just mean you both speak English, rather you both comprehend what the other one is saying. How many times have you talked to a friend, loved one or work acquaintance and, without listening to them, you have counted down the seconds before they stop talking so you can say what you need to say? This isn't listening or communicating effectively. Yet we often spend many conversations doing just this. I know I've certainly been guilty of this.

If the person comes in with the view that they have seen a handful of physiotherapists, chiropractors and exercise physiologists throughout their life and they cannot be helped, all my knowledge and expertise may be of little use to them.[37]

So, what can I do to overcome this?

I meet people where they are at.

Say someone has an injury, they have seen half a dozen people and they are hesitant. They come in and feel like all hope is lost, whatever they do is meaningless and they will suffer this pain for the rest of their days. Even with the best rehab in the world I won't be able to help unless their mind changes from a fixed state to a growth state.

To meet people where they're at, I adapt my language, mannerisms and knowledge to the person in front of me, based on the conversation I'm having or what they ask for. If they are new to pain science or basic anatomy, I won't overwhelm them with jargon and technical terms, as this will scare them and create a barrier between us. Rather I speak simply, saying that the body is resilient, that our tissues often heal without any assistance and tell them when they can expect to see results. This allows them to shift their mindset from 'I'm doomed, my life is over" to "Oh, my injury might not actually be that bad" or at bare minimum giving them a glimmer of hope.

In your life, you too will have fixed beliefs, often subconsciously; each of us has the potential for a fixed mindset.

No doubt you've entered a conversation where you thought to yourself no matter how persuasive this person is, they will not be able to change my mind. Take a moment to ponder on how your life would alter if instead you went into conversations, irrespective of the person, with an open, calm and accepting mind. You may just find that new opportunities form, new connections and doors that you otherwise would not be able to access.

Now that we have distinguished the different mindsets, fixed and growth, let's delve into why these matter – the impact of the mind in a macro sense and strategies to shift to a healthier mindset.

THE IMPACT OF MINDSET

As we have discovered, our mind is integral to how we view, engage in and overcome challenges within our lives. Mindset can give us the ability to face our fears or run from them. Much like the sympathetic and parasympathetic nervous system responses of 'fight or flight' and 'rest and digest', we have choices that will add up to favour either a fixed or growth mindset. Our choices, actions, thoughts, feelings and conditions all come with consequences.

Mental health conditions such as post-traumatic stress disorder (PTSD), anxiety, depression and schizophrenia to name a few are rampant throughout the world. These conditions can affect us as a whole, changing our physical bodies by altering our emotions, hormones and behaviours.

To give you a clear understanding of how a mental health condition or psychological condition can impact us in a physical way, here are some examples:

- Weight gain

- Increased blood pressure

- Increased risk of cancer

- Increased risk of heart disease

- Increased sensitivity to pain

- Reduced recovery

- Premature death[38]

These are not extreme examples; these are real consequences of a neglected or malnourished mindset. Such implications for our health, which extend beyond us and impact our friends, family, healthcare systems and businesses all around the world, can be avoided.

Did you know that mental conditions such as the ones listed above are the leading cause of morbidity around the world? Morbidity refers to the condition of suffering. Our mental constructs cannot and should not be ignored. The lack of care and awareness around our minds has led to countless deaths. The estimated number of people worldwide afflicted by a mental illness is slightly more than 1 in 10 at the time of writing this in 2022. You or someone you know – a friend, a family member, a client – will almost certainly experience mental health problems.

Can you change your mindset?

The short answer is yes. The long answer is yes, using neural plasticity.

NEURAL PLASTICITY

Did you know your brain is plastic? I don't mean like a plastic bottle, instead, I'm referring to our brain's ability to change, to be malleable and adapt to different circumstances. Fixed mind-sets should not really exist. Our mind is ever-changing, and the pathways and connections can develop and be undone. We know this now thanks to the study of neuroplasticity.

Within our brains and bodies exist neurons, a specific type of cell that is responsible for receiving input from the outside world. These neurons transport information to our nervous system, our muscles, and our glands. It is estimated that we have 86 billion of them in the brain.

That is 86,000,000,000. A hell of a lot of zeros! To give you some perspective, it would take nearly 32 years to count to a billion if you counted at one number per second. Wow.

This isn't even factoring in the time taken to say each number, especially the higher numbers which would take far longer. In actual fact, it would take a lot more than 32 years to count to a billion. How about doing that 86 times? Is your mind blown yet?

For those wondering, it would take about 2752 years to count that high.

Ok, enough maths.

There's a term commonly used to explain how neurons work, namely "neurons that fire together, wire together". What does this mean? Let's say we perform a specific task, like writing the alphabet. We do this over and over; the skill becomes easier and easier. We are creating strength between the specific neurons that allow us to write. These will form pathways or habits that are easily accessible to us over time, making us more efficient at performing tasks like writing. Repetition is a massive variable here. This exists in all forms of life. We are the accumulation of repeated patterns that shape our thoughts, our actions, our consciousness.

These pathways can be strengthened and weakened. Have you ever had a specific skill, such as playing an instrument, but for whatever reason you gave this up? Now, say 10 years have passed and you try to pick up this instrument and play it as well as you once did. Will you be able to? Unlikely.

The once strong neural connections of this pathway, following the principle of reversibility, have weakened. The neurons have been reallocated elsewhere to create new behaviours and improve efficiency when carrying out commonly undertaken tasks.

This construct should be understood by all that wish to affect behaviour. Creating a new pattern takes time, this goes for changing the mind and the body. If we want to learn how to speak a new language, perform a handstand or give up a toxic behaviour, we must engage in repeated actions to create the neuronal connections that allow us to form or break a habit. To repeat the quote, I used previously in the book from Aristotle, which is pertinent: "We are what we repeatedly do. Excellence, then, is not an act, but a habit."

Look to the people you admire and respect. Their qualities occur through repeated action, and you can do the same, first by changing your mindset to encourage repeated action. Consistency is the key to success in this venture.

Neuroplasticity, exercise and mindset

As mentioned, our belief, whether it's in a stimulus or a placebo, determines our success when engaging in the new behaviour. The transtheoretical model explains the phases that people can go through pre-contemplation, contemplation and planning are examples of mindset, or should I say a growth mindset. If people adopted a fixed mindset, they would not be able to transition through these stages of change.

Creating a change in behaviour must be simple: we start with a goal, determine our why and begin by taking small, active steps towards our chosen goal. There are many variables to consider when viewing mindset through the lens of creating a behaviour change to be more physically active.

It's worth mentioning here that the paradoxical nature of choice is that having too many options can lead us to make no choice at all. We should be wary of this.

Let's say you want to be healthy or healthier. The paradox of choice can often paralyse people. Where should I start? With so many components of health, it's hard to focus on one area, especially for people new to this. Is it increasing the amount of fibre in your diet, adding another HIT cardio session, cutting out smoking and drinking or improving your sleep quality? It's enough to make your head spin!

When embarking on an exercise regime and trying to promote healthier behaviours, keep it simple. As we progress, we can add layers to our regime or goals. Look at your lifestyle, and identify the lowest hanging fruit; something relatively easy to change but which will still have a big effect.

If you only get four hours of sleep per night and you are always feeling tired and lethargic, do you really think you'll be able to start exercising more all of a sudden? Unlikely. Start there and focus on sleep quality, then you'll have more energy and unconsciously move more. You may even muster the energy to actively decide to exercise!

In other words, are you focusing on the area that will have the greatest impact or are you wasting time on unhealthy habits?

Let's dig deeper into our psychology and ask why we feel the need to smoke and drink regularly, have a terrible diet and poor sleep patterns and why we aren't motivated by activity. We may uncover the culprits behind your poor behaviours, such as a lack of education or low self-efficacy or chronic work stress. Digging deeper enables us to identify how we can instigate the ripple effect, which is a small change in behaviour that can cause a cascade of changes.

This may be learning about the best way you can start moving more. Now that you have a more open mindset, you will be on the hunt for this knowledge.

Understand that less is more when it comes to behaviour change. Determine which factors will have the biggest change overall, rather than spreading yourself too thin with choice overload.

When it comes to exercise, there is a large body of research that can directly relate physiological improvements to our mindset!

Let's use the example of athletes.

We have many different forms and strains of proteins within our body. One type, the brain-derived neurotrophic factor (BDNF), particularly stands out in its relationship with our mind. This is a key protein marker for developing and maintaining the health of our neurons. It reduces and prevents the degeneration of healthy brain function and can slow the ageing process by keeping our minds sharp.[39] Cardiovascular exercises that involve rhythmical actions are essential in creating BDNF to stimulate new neurons.

Watch an athlete perform at the height of their game. What is it that makes them tick? Is it the countless hours they have spent perfecting their craft? This contributes for sure, but it's not the driving factor. What is it? Well, in my opinion, what separates the elite from the rest in any endeavour is the mindset of the individual.

These people are able to sustain the highest levels of focus and performance in their crafts due to how they've sculpted their mindset. The old saying is true that the mind gives out before the body. Train the mind to prevent this, then you will find your body excelling, making the seemingly impossible, possible.

TOOLS TO ALTER YOUR MINDSET

Techniques to craft your mind are all around you. These tools can be called upon to stem action, change your biochemistry/mood and enable you to exude power.

The first of the three tools I will discuss is changing your state.

A concept that famous life coach Tony Robbins discusses at length is his 'state'. He will use several methods to elevate this, such as priming – the act of using his breath, changing variables such as the temperature around him and chanting a mantra that shows gratitude. All top performers use a variation of this. They will have a process that enables them to access a higher version of themselves.

You can do the same. One valuable tool to directly and efficiently change your state is the anchoring effect.

FIND YOUR ANCHOR

By anchoring our emotions to a physical constraint, we create a foundation from which we can soar to our higher being. To find your anchor, first look to your passion. What makes you thrive? What's your reason for doing anything? What activity causes time to pass quickly for you? What do you daydream about? What amps you up, causing your voice, posture and emotions to change? This is your passion, and it is of utmost importance.

If you know what your passion is, you are ready to move into the anchoring phase. Now, you want to attach a word or action with the emotion you feel in your higher state. This will serve as the key to unlocking this state again in the future. Tennis superstar Rafael Nadal has a process that grounds and recentres him before each serve: he will place his hair behind his ear, touch his nose and adjust his shorts while bouncing the tennis ball. To some this appears as a strategy for time wasting; to me, it's a recalibration of his sense of self.

Determine your own anchor. This could be clicking your fingers, pulling a particular area of your skin, shouting like Ronnie Coleman "Lightweight baby" – you get the drift.

Now we come to the anchoring itself. This will take time and patience; you will need to catch yourself in a state of flow initially. When your energy is high, maybe when you are experiencing anger, love or awareness, use your physical trigger.

Repeat this a number of times, at least 15. Remember, repetition creates stronger neuronal pathways. The more we perform, the stronger the pathway. Once this connection has been established, we can utilise it at will. We all have various states in our lives; no one is perfect or primed constantly, and that's not the point. Just like we can't enjoy the sunshine without rain, we too cannot enjoy our highest state without lesser states.

These states may look like wanting to stay in and watch Netflix for the night, skipping an exercise session, or indulging in our favourite sweet treats. These states aren't the enemy at all, rather a part of you. Let yourself enjoy these moments, these lower states of yourself. It is at other times, such as presenting at an important business meeting, performing at a sporting event, wowing your partner in the bedroom, that it may be wise to call upon our higher state through our physical trigger(s).

Use this power wisely. You can't always go at it 100%. Obey the principles of rest and have periods of intensity and periods of relaxation. Use it sparingly and judiciously and watch your energy, intensity and ability to accomplish feats improve immensely.

BUILD A ROUTINE

The next key tool in allowing you to develop a powerful mindset involves your routine. Did you know your life is built on routines? Think about your current mornings – do you have a particular way of preparing yourself for the day ahead?

You might start by waking up, checking your phone, getting dressed, eating breakfast, brushing your teeth, scrolling through social media, losing track of time and rushing out the door for work.

Our routines define us. They enable us to enhance or slow down our progress. It's time to shift your conscious attention to routines. Top performers throughout the world will all have a morning routine.

My morning routine involves practising gratitude as soon as I wake up, recognising several areas of my life that I am thankful for. Then I'll get dressed, have breakfast and begin a short meditation. This allows me to relax, to tap into the parasympathetic and switch off those voices that want me to rush around doing 100 different activities. It provides me with clarity and the chance to own my day rather than being owned by it. Once I have settled into a relaxed state, I will set myself tasks for the day –crucial items that I wish to tick off my list, almost like miniature goals. That's it. This routine gives me structure, awareness and a foundation from which to continue my day. I tick these objectives off in the morning, giving me some early wins. Your routine may vary drastically from mine, and that is fine. The point is to find something that you can do to give you a strong foundation from which you can excel.

Make a mistake

An apple a day keeps the doctor away, have you ever heard of that saying? Well, I have adopted my own saying. A mistake a day keeps you on track to becoming better than yesterday.

I know what you're thinking, *Daniel, how can a mistake be a good thing*? Again, look to the greats, people that are masters in their field. Each person will credit failure for their success. Sounds contradictory, doesn't it? Failure leads to growth; it is one of the most crucial lessons anyone can learn in order to reach their dreams. Without failure, you have no sense of boundaries. Without boundaries, we don't know where our true threshold ends.

Making a mistake isn't the end of the world; in fact, it can often be the opposite. It can give you a chance to reflect, make sense of the situation and take something into your next experience. This is the power of the mistake. Our ability to use hindsight has led to advancements by leaps and bounds in technology, spiritual teachings and the human race in general.

It must be noted that context matters. The environment or way in which you make a mistake can be a matter of life or death. If you're a doctor, I'm not asking you to make some crazy leap and carry out surgery with no notion if it will work or not, as you literally may kill someone. Rather, if you make mistakes in controlled environments, ones which won't harm someone or utterly ruin your life, then they can be beneficial.

So, how can we use this to enhance our mindset? Make small, controlled mistakes and practise reflection – this could come in the form of journaling or simply recounting your day: the way you behaved, the tasks you did or didn't accomplish and so forth.

Here are a number of examples of where mistakes might occur within a controlled environment:

- Buying a co-worker a specific type of coffee without knowing if they will enjoy it or not.

- Taking an alternative route to work without the use of Google maps.

- Try listening to different genres of music while you're trying to concentrate on a task.

- Picking an outfit for the day without checking the weather first.

Mistakes are part of the human experience. No one is perfect, no matter how much some people lead you to believe they are. Even elite athletes and gurus slip up and give in to their lower beings. These controlled mistakes are easily fixable; they are designed to give you the courage to step outside your comfort zone, your boundaries, and move into your higher state.

Tell yourself that it is ok to make a mistake. Then say it again and again until you are comfortable with making mistakes. Let go of the guilt and anguish, you are human.

While I have encouraged you to make mistakes, I don't encourage you to do so without thinking about it afterwards. I guarantee you will continue to make the same mistakes until you reflect upon why you made them in the first place. Don't do this half-heartedly. Go all the way and learn from the mistake. This is when you will tap into the growth mindset and develop yourself.

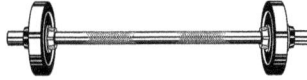

OVERVIEW

The key points I want you to take away from this chapter are:

1. The mind is powerful – its effects extend to our physical bodies. Be wary of how your beliefs might affect any stimulations (remember the placebo and nocebo effects).

2. Be aware of the psychology behind making a behavioural change.

3. Our mindset can alter our lives. Do you have a fixed or growth mindset?

4. Fixed mindsets are limiting, inflexible and absolute. There is no room for change or development.

5. Growth mindsets encourage adaptation and change. They push us forward as a society and as individuals.

6. The mind is plastic – we strengthen and weaken it through the activities we choose to engage or disengage with.

7. Utilise tools to enhance your mindset – state changing, routines and making mistakes (doctor's orders).

10

See More, Do Less

"The most important thing in communication is to hear what isn't being said."
- Peter Drucker

C ommunicating is like art. Anyone can draw or paint, but can you do this well?

To those reading this, this chapter can be viewed in multiple streams. For a practitioner, this will be applicable for coaching. For the general population, this is more applicable to daily life — business, relationships and learning.

Knowing how to explain and/or demonstrate the point you are trying to make is a skill, a valuable one at that, but it is not the only skill required to be a good communicator. This chapter will largely focus on intrapersonal skills: the way we communicate, our body language, how to listen to someone and our ability to connect and empathise.

Think of a mentor, someone you admire in your life. What qualities do they possess? Why are you drawn to this particular person?

A well-rounded communicator has the ability to convey their message in different ways. Take 100 people and tell them the same message, we may get up to 100 different interpretations. Why is this? People are different. Their goals, previous experiences, injury histories, mindsets, ability to comprehend will vary vastly. Do not fall into the trap of applying the same concept or model to each person you meet. From a clinical perspective, this may look like seeing somebody with knee pain and just giving them a glute exercise because that had helped someone in the past. In doing so, you move away from a client-centred approach in which you are listening and understanding them – their fears, goals, lifestyles and patterns that have led them to seeking your help. An exceptional coach will explore the various pathways that can lead to the end goal. They will adapt to the needs of the client, altering the language they use, the sensations they stimulate and the way they provide feedback.

Everyone will have experienced a teacher they did not gel with, someone in their lives that they relied upon for information or a certain skill yet were put off so gave up, switched off and branded them a bad influence. What was it about this person that made them a bad teacher? Was it their tone of voice, the way they explained the content, the fact that they read information to you word for word and didn't care to elaborate? One size does not fit all in the area of communicating, unfortunately. Intelligence is multi-faceted, we all learn differently than the next person and favour specific types of teaching over others. Become a better communicator and start leading yourself towards a better life through accountability, responsibility and clarity.

LEARNING ARCHETYPES

Within the constructs of learning exist several distinctive ways we engage with information. The ways I will follow relate to the popular VARK model, which involves auditory, visual, reading

and writing and kinaesthetic types of learners.[40] These archetypes of learning mirror our senses (hearing, sight, smell, taste
and touch). Some rely more than others on certain senses – we
are all different. Knowing yourself in this regard will allow you
to understand your strengths and weaknesses as a learner.

AUDITORY LEARNING

This refers to the human sense of hearing. These archetypes prefer to record or read out loud their material and create acronyms
or mnemonic phrases to assist with their learning. Auditory
learners prefer not to take notes and instead listen to the material
being presented to them. As a coach, we may recommend a
particular podcast for them to listen to, the demands of the task
at hand should be explained in detail and conversations should
be undertaken to elicit understanding.

VISUAL LEARNING

The visual learner relies more on infographics, pictures and im-
ages that explain to them what words cannot. Do you think
all paintings look the same? Can you tell the difference in their
styles? Maybe you aren't well-versed in artistic styles, but you
may still be this type of learner if you prefer tables, graphics or
pictures over paragraphs. We can apply this to coaching through
illustrating the goals, habits and expectations we set for our
clients through colour coding, graphs and flow charts to explain
what actions are required to achieve their desired change and
exhibit their progress over time.

READING AND WRITING

This brings me back to when I was in Year 1 at school and told to
repeatedly write certain sentences over and over, tediously filling
exercise books with words and phrases so I could remember how

to write them. This is a form of repetition. Rote learning is a common phrase used to describe this style, where we aim to learn the content through essentially copying and pasting the information. You will see this flourishing within the schooling system: people that love to take notes after reading a particular text, then later revising through the same protocol of reading and rewriting. For this archetype, a coach may provide written summaries of their results as opposed to a graph, they will encourage discussion via email so the learner can reflect on their thoughts and feelings about the quality of their session and any questions they may have.

KINAESTHETIC

Kinaesthetic relates to the act of doing, touching and feeling our way through the material. These people will excel at hands-on experience. I am in this category; I learn best once I have tried an activity for myself. Let's take carpentry, for example. Someone can show me how to do it, they can tell me how to do it and I can read books about carpentry techniques, but until I begin experimenting with the skills, tools and handling involved, I will not fully grasp it. These types of people simply need to perform the skill. If your client is in this category, it's best when teaching them a movement to let them use their hands, feet or whatever part of the body to feel the position. They will understand and learn through what their touch receptors are telling them.

Do you feel you fit into more than one of these learning archetypes? This is entirely possible as well. We are adaptative by nature, and therefore have the potential to learn using different learning styles. Keep this in your mind when creating the best environment for either you or a client to change. Applying this model towards someone's individual style may allow something once thought of as difficult to become tolerable.

How do we discover our bias?

While I mentioned above that we will possess an affinity to learn in each of the four archetypes, the rate and effectiveness at which we learn is vastly different.

A simple way to learn your preferred method is to try each one: you'll soon discover which style you are most drawn to. There are also a number of questionnaires available to highlight which category we favour. Research and reflect on your own style. The content within this book may start you on your path to discovery: maybe you relate more with the diagrams used throughout the book, maybe some of the examples I used allowed you to retain and picture the events in a clear way. You might find yourself wishing this was turned into an audiobook or podcast to further explain concepts. Pay attention and your archetype will appear. Be aware of what you are drawn to, as this will enhance your productivity, comprehension and ability to use this information in a practical way.

Intrapersonal skills

As a coach, what we don't say or do can be just as important as what we do say or do. Equally, how we present information is important when educating, inspiring and conveying meaning. There are a variety of verbal, physical and auditory methods which utilise the body's senses that can be used when giving feedback to help us and those around us to get the message. This comes through our dominant communication style, the body language we project, the words we use, our tone and how we can listen and show empathy for the people in front of us.

COMMUNICATION IS KEY

Communication is essential. Let me take you back to our hunter-gather days. We, as human beings, had to communicate in order to successfully hunt and conquer our prey. We had to work in unison, delegate roles, use weapons and tools and create a plan if we were to eat, to live. Communication has driven the human race forward, with the ability to speak being considered a key difference separating us from the rest of the animal kingdom. Without communication we could not teach, pass down information from generation to generation and build upon our previously learned lessons.

Communication is a fundamental life skill. The ability to communicate, spread knowledge from one place or person to the next, can be the difference between friendship or loneliness, being employed or unemployed, being understood or misperceived. We use communication throughout our lives to inform, express, influence and convey our thoughts, feelings, emotions and perspectives to those around us.

It's no different with health and fitness. We communicate with ourselves daily. No doubt you've told yourself, "One more rep" or said, "Nah, I'll skip legs today".

The act of communicating positively or negatively with yourself can ultimately lead to success or failure in reaching your goals.

DID YOU KNOW YOUR BODY CAN TALK?

Have you ever considered how you look to those around you? I know I have! I used to do this in a superficial, anxious way. "What is this person thinking of me?", "Are they judging me?" etc. As I have grown, I have learnt to be more conscious of body language.

Our nonverbal actions, the way we communicate with our body, is just as important as what we say. Body language refers to our facial expressions, how we gesture and hold ourselves, as well as the way we move our eyes and hands.

When communicating with people, the nonverbal is estimated to account for a whopping 70 to 90% of the message we convey, more so than language, tone and any other form of communication we use!

Let's use an example to demonstrate this. We have the first salesperson, Maria, trying to sell you a new product that can supposedly change your life.

Maria stumbles over to you with a blank expression on her face and introduces herself. She doesn't look comfortable, she is slouched, she doesn't offer to shake your hand, she doesn't even attempt to make eye contact with you, and she's shifting around so much that it's starting to make you nervous.

Lucy, the second salesperson, confidently approaches you. Lucy makes eye contact, has a warm smile on her face and gives a friendly wave. She offers her hand in a welcoming way when she reaches you. She stands tall, maintains eye contact and makes you feel comfortable immediately, so you are receptive to what she is saying.

Now, both salespeople said the same thing and are selling the same product, but there were two different outcomes. What changed? With both salespeople, before they even opened their mouths, you were unconsciously watching them; you were breaking down and measuring your ability to trust them through their body language. Our body language is the way we walk, the softness or hardness of our face, the distance we create and the attention we demand through our gaze. Maria failed to create a warming environment. She was distant, shifty and unwelcoming, so she didn't make the sale.

Have you met people like this? I'm sure we all have. We gain insight into somebody's character by watching the way they move. Do they hold themselves with grace, strength and charisma or are they reserved, hesitant and zestless?

LANGUAGE USED

If we lose touch with ourselves, our direction and our purpose, we may find ourselves behaving in ways that just aren't us. It's as if we are speaking another language, one that is incomprehensible to us.

Throughout my life, I have learned the language of human anatomy and physiology, which I have sprinkled throughout this book. Some of the words I have used may not make sense, leading me to the conclusion I have not done a good enough job of conveying my message to you, the reader. The language used within any profession is essential for better understanding.

In the health profession, we may utilise terms such as sagittal plane, flexion and extension, inhibitions and activations to name a few. The ability of a good coach lies not in knowing this language, but rather understanding how to express what they mean in layman's terms. If I told you I wanted you to segmentally flex each joint in your body starting from your cervical spine, through your thoracic spine and lumbar spine until you have a uniform spinal curve at your thoracolumbar junction, with your centre of gravity reaching end range at the distal metatarsal phalangeal joints so I can assess your functional range of motion within multiple segments, what would you say or do? Sigh, probably.

Now, if I told you to try and bend forward through your spine starting from your neck and aim to touch your toes, would you understand?

I have said the exact same things, the first to a clinician, the other to a client. Whether explaining a concept at work, giving advice to a friend or telling off our children, we must be conscious of the language we use.

People might nod their head and smile to give you the idea that they understand what you are asking of them, and in some cases they might, but others will have no idea what you are saying, and you will be none the wiser.

Do you ever dig deeper when communicating, whether that's with your partner, your employer or employee, even your local barista?

One useful technique is to ask yourself questions throughout your conversation.

1. Are they actually listening to me? If I have asked a question of them and I get a blank stare and start hearing crickets in the background, I know I have failed to engage this person. They have stopped listening, misunderstood and the point I was aiming to get across evaporates into nothingness.

2. Could they relay this information back to me? Our ability to comprehend depends on how we break up the given information into bite-sized pieces that we can understand. If a person cannot relay the information back to you, do you think they understand it?

Each person has their own unique style to articulate themselves. The language they use, their jargon, phrases and terms, can be vastly different, whether it's a tradesman, doctor or musician. ,.

You get the point. Adapt your language to those you engage with.

This doesn't mean mastering the lingo for every profession out there unless you are that way inclined. Rather, I am asking you to think outside of the box when communicating with those around you; meet people halfway. This may look like trying to understand the slang or terms they frequently use and adjusting your language to match. This can help to build rapport and develop your relationships with people, in essence making you not only a better communicator but a better person.

In the same way we adapt our language to others, we can teach others to do the same. When striking up a conversation, giving context goes a long way.

If I simply tell a client to pull their ribs down and leave it at that, they will most likely just give me a blank stare. We need to explain the meaning behind the language we are using. Show them, break it down for them, and adapt your language as they progress through their training. Rather than simply saying pull your ribs down, show them where the ribs are, how to know if the ribcage is moving and why we care in the first place, for example, the ribs should expand up and outwards when breathing in, and pull down and inwards when breathing out.

Another example of context is how we talk to children. Have you ever been stuck in the middle of two kids having an argument? They will rush through their version of events, spitting it out as quickly as possible. So, what should we do? Rush to conclusions and reprimand the person who was slower to tell their story? Not ideally. A better approach is to slow them both down, get each side of the story (ideally separately) from the beginning and then begin to process and make sense of the situation. From here you have the context to be able to make a well-informed decision about what action if any, needs to be taken. Without the context, we simply have a breakdown in communication and will disconnect rather than connect with the person in front of us.

Do you test how effectively you use language?

We all like to think we are good at something until we are told otherwise. Communicating is no different. We aren't born perfect at communicating, it is a skill that needs to be mastered. I've met teenagers that are better at articulating their point than a 50-year-old, purely because they have taken the time to develop this skill. Find some objective measures in your everyday conversations, for example how often you have to repeat yourself, how often you get a blank stare or an exclamation of "What?!" If you find yourself getting frustrated because people are difficult to talk to, then remember this old saying: "If you meet an asshole, then they are an asshole. If everyone you meet is an asshole, then you are the asshole."

This applies to communicating. If you think everyone is terrible at talking to you or engaging with you, it is likely the problem lies with you and your style of communicating. The better you get, the easier those conversations will become.

Tone of voice

Our tone of voice is a big deal. We can say the same words, and use the same language, yet the person in front of us can perceive them in completely different ways. Have you ever had someone say to you they don't like the tone of your voice? Maybe your partner, parent or friend felt offended or experienced a negative emotion due to the way you said something? You may have even had good intentions and strung together a nice sentence, yet your tone of voice did not match what you were saying. The tone of your voice refers to its pitch and depth, whether you are enthusiastic or robotic, if we convey any emotions like anger, sadness, joy.

It is a crucial variable that can lead to effective or ineffective communication between two people.

Read the following sentence aloud:

"Hi, how are you?"

Now, repeat this phrase and match it to each of the following scenarios:

- Meeting someone you are excited to see

- Meeting someone you hate

- Working in a retail store and greeting a new customer

- As above, but while you're in a rush during the holiday period

- Saying this when you are exhausted

- Saying this when you are drunk

For each of these scenarios, we have said the same phrase but probably in a different tone. You may have been loud, expressive and inviting in some of these scenarios, with others you may have seem uninterested, lacklustre and even intimidating.

Being aware of how we say what we say can be the difference between appearing interested or uninterested; between you getting respect or someone thinking you are full of yourself.

ACTIVE LISTENING

"Excuse me, can you repeat that?"

We have two ears and one mouth, yet the majority of us speak more than we listen.

Do you take the time to listen to the person in front of you, or are you simply waiting for your turn to speak?

If you are an active listener, then you will be able to relay what someone has said back to them in a meaningful way. Have you ever spoken to someone who tries to finish your sentences? Does it leave you frustrated when they always end up saying the wrong words? This person does not actively listen. In contrast, you may have someone that you can talk to, your confidant, who is patient, stays quiet and gives input when needed. Not just any input though; active listening often involves reciting what the person has said to you in your own way, giving advice and building upon the conversation.

Active listening involves giving the person your undivided attention and maintaining eye contact, not fidgeting and looking like you are trying to escape the conversation. This gives the person the sense of being understood, supported and, most importantly, listened to. Now, who doesn't want that?

Active listening also involves being able to relay what has been said to you, in a way that is meaningful to you. Rather than jumping to conclusions and misinterpreting the situation, you will instead wait for the person to finish speaking. Then, you may recite what they said in your own words, something beginning with "I think what you're trying to say is ..." This is not to assume, rather it allows the person to clarify if needs be.

Active listening is an invaluable tool for creating connections. Giving someone the space to feel listened to is powerful. If you find yourself surrounded by quiet people, become one of them or ask more open-ended, inviting questions and you will see them open up.

CONNECTION AND EMPATHY

Understanding, connecting and practising empathy within our conversations with people are the qualities of an exceptional communicator.

Have you ever been into a doctor's surgery, sat down next to the doctor only for them to hurry you along with your problem, barely making eye contact before sending you out the door? Did you connect with this person? Unlikely.

In my own clinical experience, I have seen and worked with highly knowledgeable practitioners, ones that know the ins and outs of their chosen speciality, yet their clientele did not keep them busy. Why was this? It wasn't for a lack of patients, it wasn't because they didn't know how to help the person they were seeing, rather they failed to connect. They did not create buy-in, rapport, a supportive environment for the person they were seeing. Often people will cease to care about what you know or have to say unless you make it meaningful to them; if you're a monotone robot with no ability to connect with a person through a mutual understanding, good luck at helping them.

Practising empathy and the previous aspects of communication we have discussed will lead to meaningful relationships with those around you. This is a crucial aspect for your overall health. The social constructs you engage with can empower you or bury you. Employing these strategies will enable you to see which relationships are worth harvesting and nourishing and which are worth leaving and moving on from.

Types of memory

We know that throughout our brain exist neurons, a collection of cells that create pathways for every action and thought we have. Within the context of learning a new skill, pattern or movement, there are stages much like the stages of change. As we become more proficient with a new task, some faster than others, we pass through three distinct stages: cognitive, associative and autonomous.

The student, the teacher, the master

Learning this model of skill acquisition and its three stages (cognitive, associative and autonomous) is vital as it differentiates how we administer exercise progressions and regressions, the language we use and the stimulus we give ourselves or our clients to continue making progress. We must be familiar with the key variables within each archetype of the learning curve, as this will give us a rationale, guidance and ensure our programmes are effective.

Cognitive

Within the cognitive stage, we are fresh, new to the skill or task at hand. This skill will be very difficult at first, lots of errors and mistakes are likely to occur and we will place a large emphasis on the internal characteristics.

Think back to learning to ride a push bike for the first time. If you haven't tried this, give it a go! What you will find or remember from trying to ride is falling off a lot, learning balance and coordination, and focusing on holding on to the handlebars for dear life (or maybe this was just me ...). In any case, you would not have been aware of your surroundings, the cars and people walking past. In other words, you focused on the internal environment (balance, trying to hold on and stay upright) compared to the external environment (the cars, people and outside noises or hazards).

Within the cognitive stage, we often see rapid progression. Much like in the gym, we can reap significant adaptations in a short amount of time through our nervous system becoming more efficient and the growth of our muscular system. In the context of learning a new movement, we aren't concerned with the weight.

Let's apply this to doing squats at the gym. When we first squat, we aren't going to load up 100kg and go for gold. Instead, we may just use our body weight. The focus for this squat could be ensuring you can control your lumbopelvic region during the descent, maintain good contact with the floor through using the entirety of your feet or controlling the movement through the desired range of motion.

People within this stage will need constant reassurance, positive feedback and advice on how to improve and correct their errors. Be patient and mindful of the learning curve; it is very easy for people within this stage to get frustrated and want to give up. Remember, after a period of rain comes the sunshine.

ASSOCIATIVE

To explain the associative stage, let's revisit our bike-riding example. When we move into this part of our learning, we start to look up from our hands and the pedals and look at the world around us – shift from the internal to the external. Here, we have developed the ability to control the fundamental demands of the task and we can venture into new areas to conquer. The associative phase will require a more specific approach than the cognitive stage.

This specific approach involves 'deliberate practice', meaning we must break down the skill and focus on specific sub-components to improve. Keep in mind, you will still make mistakes in the associative stage as you learn new areas of the skill, sport or movement. This may look like developing accuracy when throwing a ball as opposed to just being able to throw a ball. Accuracy will take time to develop.

The associative stage, from a coaching perspective, is where we as trainers choose whether to give feedback or decide if the person is capable of doing that themselves. We are still very essential within this stage, but I recommend being circumspect about how and when exactly you give feedback around their results and errors; we want to promote independence and growth rather than keeping someone reliant on us.

Autonomous

Who's your favourite athlete, musician, artist or entertainer?

These people will all have something in common, something that has allowed them to get to the top of their speciality and excel at the task in front of them.

Any guesses what that might be?

They are autonomous. They flow, have a certain energy that allows them to complete complex tasks with relative ease. Think back to the concept of anchoring ourselves to a higher state. These people are exceptional at finding this state and maintaining it throughout their performance. This has developed through a combination of skill and hard work and, as we know, rituals and triggers. They have dedicated themselves to their chosen field; time, energy, learning and failure were some of the key components that have allowed them to reach a stage of autonomy. Not all people engaging within a skill will reach this stage; many will stay at the associative stage.

Autonomous people have mastered the internal and external. Thinking about the skill is no longer required, they instead act on impulse. It is an unconscious pattern; one they have created through strong neuronal connections of repeated exposure. They are able to give themselves their own feedback, reflecting on what they did well and not so well within their performance. They are able to adapt and customise their approach if they choose to.

This stage presents a choice between contentment, plateau and stagnation (fixed state) or continued growth, striving to improve our skills to our fullest capability.

Take the example of speaking in your first language. Let's assume this is English, as you are currently reading this book. Now, we may all be adept at speaking English, but are we in the autonomous stage? We know how to speak, but can we speak clearly in a structured, coherent manner? Are we able to do this effortlessly and string complex words together to make a point crystal clear, with correct pronunciation and pauses? For many of us, this is not the case; we may stumble or slur a word here and there. The English language is vast and complex. How much of the terminology – oxymorons, juxtaposition, hyperbole, etc. – do you have within your arsenal of communicating? Many of us are adept at speaking but not masters of the English language. We can choose to enhance our English skills or remain content with our current abilities.

The three stages are intertwined and abide by the law of reversibility. Injury, ageing and the endeavour to learn new components of a mastered skill can be humbling and take us back to being novices. We can then layer more complex patterns on top of one another through the different stages of learning.

Quite often, our patterns can lead us to injury, so we must relearn the fundamentals and change how we do the skill in the first place. Remember that we constantly compensate and adopt analgesic patterns to take the load off the injured areas. If left to our own devices, this can drastically change how we perform a skill, leading us to regress rather than progress.

Time adheres to the principle of reversibility. We can gain back what we lost relatively quickly after having time off, but there is a definite drop off in our ability to engage in the skill required. We also have that annoying problem of ageing. As we age, we slow down, our cells become less productive, our ability to react decreases and our ability to act at our prime can fade.

Lastly, the process of learning new skills means making lots of errors, and we will be placed out of our comfort zones once again.

A coach like myself, for instance, will come across many different personality types and have the ability to adapt our way of communicating to encourage choice and appropriate feedback. I may, however, want to better express empathy and understanding, or maybe change my style of coaching. To do this I'll need to go through the process of learning, making mistakes and doubting myself. I may seek guidance from another coach to help me develop.

Each of these examples can lead us towards a transition in ourselves, our abilities and what we once thought of as absolute. Change is encouraged; for me, a constant state of uncomfortableness and flux allows me to propel my knowledge, growth and ability to be the best version of myself. Do you seek out uncomfortable situations? Or are you happy staying the same?

The message I want to get across within this chapter has been to constantly approach situations from different perspectives. Apply this to some basic mathematics. We can get to six by adding three to three, taking two from eight or multiplying two by three. People are the same. We need to consistently arm ourselves with new knowledge, adding to the range of tools at our disposal.

You should regularly test your ability to communicate your message. Say it to yourself in different ways, try and explain concepts to your friends and family, people with no background knowledge and experts on the subject at hand. This is how we learn, grow and ultimately enhance our skill set to enable us to live a life of meaning, purpose and constant growth.

We should demand this level from ourselves. This is for all areas of life.

11

What to Do & What Not to Do

"We are what we repeatedly do, excellence, then, is not an act, but a habit." - Aristotle

L ights, camera, action.

You are Shrek.

You have just been told you are at the beginning of a dangerous quest; you have no knowledge of what to do and hardly an inkling of where to go.

In the beginning, it's just you vs. the world, with no one to guide or help you. No instructions or cheat sheets. Just you. This quest will challenge you, physically, emotionally, and psychologically.

Nervous yet?

Now let's change some details, and brighten the mood with the song "From Misery to Happiness": *I'm on my way from misery to happiness today, uh huh, uh huh, uh huh, uh huh.*

Yes, it's still just you, you're still on a quest; only now you're longing for a healthier lifestyle not a prince or princess (or maybe both?).

What do you do? Where do you start? Who can you enlist to help you?

You just have the outcome – the goal of being a healthier you or at least a subset of that goal.

If Shrek had structure, a cheat sheet, or better yet a giant map that showed a range of obstacles and how to easily safeguard against them, do you think he would have succeeded?

Yes.

Although it wouldn't be very entertaining, it would have been a much simpler journey.

So, what about you?

Would you like structure, an idea of what to do and not to do?

Well, keep reading and watch your quest get a whole lot easier.

Whenever we begin a new task, the same question will always arise: what do I need to do to accomplish this task?

Enter, structure.

The structure can come in the form of a programme, an action plan, or an outline of your day. Structure gives you a blueprint of the important variables, a short guide that you can refer to throughout your quest to ensure you are on the right path.

Plot twist time …

We are going to start with what not to do. When mapping out our plan, think of exclusion criteria: those deadly obstacles like a dragon that we must avoid at all costs.

You open up a scroll and all it says is "Walk". Is this a sufficient plan?

VARIABLE I: LACK OF GOAL SETTING

Are you at the start of your quest? Maybe you want to move or train more? The first pitfall often starts with people getting a surge of motivation. A classic time for this is at the start of a new year. "New year, new me" can lead to starting towards that goal you've been dreading the previous year of going to a gym. What do you think the success rate of new year resolutions is?

At six months, research suggests only 46% of people are staying true to their resolutions.

This is massive! Imagine you started your quest with 100 people; after six months, 54 of your comrades have died. Damn.

Have you ever thought about why these new year resolutions often fail within the first few weeks?

It'd due to a lack of clarity. They missed the key variable of goal setting.

Remember that old saying: "Fail to prepare, prepare to fail." This concept is incredibly relevant to you and your quest: fail to prepare where you are going on your quest, and you'll be hard pressed to reach your destination successfully. You may as well quit now and save yourself from getting crushed by a dragon in a castle or, worse, becoming a statistic!

Now, I know new year's resolutioners can get a bad rap. It's not a bad thing to want to start being healthy. I am an advocate of people moving and staying active; and I give credit to anybody who decides they want to make a change to become a healthier

WHAT TO DO & WHAT NOT TO DO   181

person. The missing piece in achieving this, however, is the execution.

You and me have both seen our fair share of people who what to complete a task, yet, much like the millions of people who have a grandiose new year's resolution, fall back into their old habits within a week, maybe a month.

Failing to prepare is failing to set goals.

Goal setting will give you direction, purpose and intent to create effective, efficient and appropriate programmes. Without a goal, turning up to complete a workout is like buying a Ferrari and leaving the fuel tank empty ... looks good, but you aren't going anywhere.

I will delve into the nuances, pitfalls and the nitty gritty of goal setting in Chapter 2.

VARIABLE 2: INDIVIDUALISATION

Now we know you need a decent goal to anchor you and give direction in your quest.

Let's say you stumble across another scroll; you open this one up and it says "Avoid danger". Seriously, who writes these scrolls?

This is akin to surfing the internet, stumbling across a training programme and thinking it is perfect for you.

Such a programme was not written for you. It doesn't understand your background – injuries, broken bones, medical conditions, time constraints, goals, lifestyle. You get the point.

Now, you can get a generic programme off the internet and still get results. This is still better (in most cases) than just training with no goal in mind or structured programming.

It's not until you engage in a programme that is written for you, goal orientated and appropriate for someone with your medical history that you truly see significant results.

VARIABLE 3: BALANCE

Ever heard of any of the following sayings?

- "Every day is chest day."

- "I skipped leg day."

- "I'm just going to train my mirror muscles."

- "I just want a party pump."

These are just a few terms that get thrown around. The variable missing from these types of programmes is balance.

An example? Performing five chest exercises vs. two back exercises.

Now, if we consider the point above in the context of individualisation, we can make a case for favouring this imbalance of five chest vs. two back exercises.

- You may be recovering from a chest injury and require development of this area due to atrophy from a lack of movement.

- You may be a bodybuilder who wants a specialised programme to develop your chest muscles.

- Or you may be someone who just wants a big chest and doesn't care about your back.

For the majority of you reading this, though, you will need balance. So, using our above scenario, we would instead look to even the odds, so to speak, and perform five chest exercises and five back exercises.

While we are talking about the gym here, in a broader context of reaching your goals balance is still of utmost importance.

Let's say you set yourself a financial goal of earning a certain amount for the financial year. Now you have a clear goal and your plan is to simply work more hours per week to achieve this goal.

You're ticking boxes so far: you have structure and a clear goal that's individual to you.

Only, you have neglected balance. To achieve this goal of earning more money by working more hours, you need to sacrifice time from elsewhere.

Unfortunately, we only have 168 hours in the week, and this doesn't change. So, we must sacrifice something from our week: maybe you start skipping social events, family time or engaging in healthy behaviours like exercising or sports.

This is where it starts to get unbalanced. As we will delve into this book, you'll discover health is more than just merely the physical. Health is an accumulation of the physical, the mental and the emotional. To be truly healthy, we must aim for a balanced lifestyle.

VARIABLE 4: APPROPRIATENESS

You, yes you, the one reading this book. Let me ask you a question. Are you new to training?

If so, you are classified as a novice or someone with less than 6 months of experience. Novice is a boring name so from henceforth, you will be known as 'Tenderfoot'.

Now, Tenderfoot, are you trying to perform incredible feats in your first programme?

These might look like the following:

- Squatting 100kg without ever having squatted before.

- Running a marathon with no prior training.

- Jumping over a car speeding at you (ok, maybe not this one).

Now, these are all extreme examples, I know. But you get the point. They demonstrate that people have a tendency to overdo it in their Tenderfoot days.

We need to make our programming appropriate for us.

If you are a Tenderfoot, you can get away with a lot less. The phrase "work smarter, not harder" was coined for you.

Let's look at a scenario to figure out our appropriateness.

We have two people, a Tenderfoot and an Olympic athlete – someone who has dedicated their life to their sport.

Now, should we:

A) Give them the same stimulus

B) Give them stimuli based on their individual wants, goals and needs

C) Skip the question because we don't know the answer

Drum roll ...

Hopefully, you answered A.

Just joking, it's B.

The same programme would not be appropriate due to a difference in training age (the number of years you have trained).

Training age dictates how much we require to continue to see growth.

As we begin our endeavours, we need very little, as literally everything is a stimulus for us.

As we progress in our quest and become more experienced, we become, shall we say, battle-hardened. This allows us to conquer earlier obstacles with ease, so now we require a bigger, harder obstacle e.g., more training volume or intensity to continue to see improvements.

HERE'S A QUICK RULE OF THUMB

Novice (Up to six months) – You can see results with minimal stimulus e.g., in a gym-training context, one set per working muscle per week

Intermediate (six months to two years) – You need more stimulus, you battle-hardened soldier! You now need roughly 10 sets per working muscle per week.

Advanced (two years plus) – You've been doing this for a while. You know the ropes and now require roughly 10-20 sets per working muscle per week.

Using this as a snapshot, we can determine the appropriate exposure at the time to whatever stimulus we are after.

You can think of this as like driving a car. When you first get behind the wheel, you're anxious. There are a million things to check – mirrors, car seat, steering wheel height, where the hell is the pedal, what the hell is a clutch and so on.

It's overwhelming. Now, flash forward to you getting your provisional plates – you know the ropes, maybe you've even got the car set up the way you like it, you can drive and it's not so overwhelming.

Now, we have our advanced soldier, let's call him Jean. Jean is a pro, in fact, Jean is so good he can go into what is called auto-pilot mode in which he requires very little concentration on what he is doing. Why? He just has that much experience, so much exposure to the act of driving that he can switch off. If Jean wants to improve his skills, he might have to take a further driving test; simply telling him to speed up and slow down isn't enough for him anymore. Jean wants to do high-speed chases, hard manoeuvres, and death-defying acts, so he needs more stimulus or training.

VARIABLE 5: TOO MUCH, TOO EARLY

I'm with you. There is so much information out there it's enough to make your head explode. Where do we start?

Well, if I'm still talking to you, Tenderfoot, I'd say this. Keep it simple.

I'm going to assume you've run before. Now, I want you to think about a race, maybe you had to run 3km in primary school for a cross country. Doing too much, too early will give you an early lead, but, like the fable of the hare and tortoise, you will also burn out quicker. Hell, you might not even finish the race if you peak too early!

This is common when starting out, as we found with our new year's resolutioners: we may have a surge of energy, leading us to want to complete everything at once. Often, this surge of energy is short-lived: we go to the gym and use every machine we can see, maybe even stop by another gym on the way home and repeat the process because you are just pumped with energy!

Flash forward to the next day and you can't move a single one of the 700 muscles in your body without it hurting. You went too hard, too early.

Keep it simple when starting.

This is the best advice I can give you. Don't jump from programme to programme, trying the coolest and craziest methods out there. Start small, build a decent foundation and go from there. Probably not what you wanted to hear, right?

Take it from me, someone who was once where you are, reading through everything and wanting to get big and strong as fast as possible. Little did I know, less was more.

My sessions used to last for hours, leaving me limping out of the gym, dreading the muscle soreness that would run over me like a fire engine the next day.

Now, this can be fun and I actually encourage you to perform some crazy sessions here and there, to add some variety and move away from your comfort zone ... but further down the track.

First, get some much-needed experience and learn good mechanical techniques– break it down, understand the components and build it back up.

Once adept in this, you can look to conquer other similar skills using the same process; before you know it, you won't be looking in the mirror at Tenderfoot, you'll be looking in the mirror and seeing Jean.

WHAT VARIABLES DOES A GOOD PROGRAMME HAVE?

You guessed it, everything we just talked about!

A good programme will be specific to you. It will be goal-oriented, it will be appropriate, individualised, balanced and hit that fine line between too much and not enough.

Put your hand up if you want this programme! Ok, I can't actually see your hand; you probably look weird now, so feel free to drop it back down.

One thing I am yet to touch upon, but is a factor I deem of great importance, is adherence. I often say to my clients and patients that I could write them the best individualised, balanced, goal-oriented programme that they have ever laid their eyes on. This programme could be perfect for them in every way, shape and form and yet useless if they don't stick to it.

This book does not have any secret answers, it is not riddled with magic solutions to your problems. Rather, this is going to entail a systematic approach that you can use for your training. The biggest step after receiving this education is actually applying the new-found knowledge consistently.

After all what is knowledge if we do not put it into practice?

Just like our new year's resolution goal setters earlier, people will often fail in their quest for a healthier life through exercise, or any goal for that matter, because they don't stick to the task.

Adherence could be its own chapter in this book.

It is of utmost importance to be adherent when achieving anything in life.

AN EXAMPLE OF POOR ADHERENCE

There was once a personal trainer (PT) who took on a new client named Jack. Now, Jack comes with goals of gaining x amount of muscle, trying to get that summer shred. The personal trainer says Jack will need to resistance train three or four times per week, hit certain protein targets and adhere to all the other

advice they give him. Jack starts off strong, his motivation is high and he sticks to every piece of advice given to him. Great start, Jack.

However, everyday commitments of work, paying bills, social-ising, etc. start getting in the way, and Jack has to cancel a few sessions with his personal trainer. Jack also has some exams com-ing up, and he has been so focused on studying that he misses a few meals here and there and doesn't track his diet regularly anymore.

It's now been around six weeks of training and Jack and his PT are checking in, doing measurements to look at his progress so far. Jack becomes disheartened because his muscles aren't bulging out of his shirt. Jack starts to question this personal trainer and asks why isn't he getting results.

The PT states that it takes approximately eight to 12 weeks for muscle growth to become noticeable and that gaining muscle can actually be quite a slow process, one that requires patience and adherence. Jack is not happy with this answer and decides to stop using this PT as he assumes he isn't good at his job.

Is Jack correct? In this scenario, no.

Personal trainers can take a lot of crap in this industry; it is very results-based for a large demographic of clients. If they do not see results quickly, they will seek to blame their assigned trainer. Now, in the above scenario, Jack failed to adhere to the guidelines recommended by his PT. It wasn't on purpose; Jack had every intention of getting shredded, but life got in the way.

No doubt you are in the same boat as Jack: we all have events, situations that emerge and commitments that will continually arise. If we think back to the things we have quit in our lives, like playing an instrument, sports, or learning a new language, why did we quit? Was it because we didn't see results or didn't feel we were good enough? Take a moment to reflect on these circumstances throughout your life, and ask yourself how adherent you were to the tasks you quit and those things in which you succeeded.

Were you like Jack? Did you fail to undertake the fundamental tasks required to attain results?

Now, there are many reasons for low adherence. I want this to be food for thought, a bit of self-reflection- if you will.

Next time you try a new skill – it doesn't even need to be health or fitness related – I want you to check how adherent you are to the constraints that are required for results.

First, identify what you want to achieve.

Then, ask yourself how you can objectively measure the results e.g., comparing how many sessions you are supposed to train in a week vs. how many you actually do.

Keep going until you reach your goal or fail. If you fail, look through your metrics and see what let you down!

So far, we have started to identify some common themes of a good structure. Something to start you on your journey. I want to now dig deeper into this and break down further what each of these variables are, how we can use them, and why it's so important for you and me to abide by them.

12

Why, Why, and a Dash of Why.

"The thing about goals is that living without them is a lot more fun, in the short run. It seems to me, though, that ,who lead, who grow and who make an impact... those people have goals." - Seth Godin

Coach: "It's time to set your goals, the reason you have decided to train today. Through our conversation, I would like to uncover both short- and long-term goals, your current perceived limitations as well as your priorities."

Client: "That sounds great! Well, the reason I came here today is because I want to lose weight."

Coach: "You want to lose weight? Ok, so why is this important to you?"

Client: "I want to lose weight because of how I look."

Coach: "Ok, what is wrong with how you look?"

Client: "Well, I feel like I can't keep up with my daily activities anymore, and when I walk past mirrors, I will sometimes catch a glimpse of myself and become frustrated and upset."

Coach: "I see, so let's start with your frustration. why have you become frustrated with your appearance?"

Client: "I used to be a lot skinnier before I had kids. Since then, I have let myself go and become increasingly less motivated the longer I leave it."

Coach: "So, why today? What gave you the motivation to walk in?"

Client: "I am fed up. I need to change; I need to get back to who I was. I don't like the person I have become."

Coach: "Who was this person?"

Client: "They were strong, confident, bubbly! I used to be known for my charisma, and I miss who I was. I want my child to see that side of me, I want my husband to see that I'm still me."

Coach: "This is a massive step walking in here today then, you should be proud of yourself! It sounds like you are ready to make a real impact on your lifestyle and health!"

Client: "Yes, definitely!"

Coach: "Tell me about your energy. You mentioned that you are struggling with your everyday activities?"

Client: "Well, you know, the everyday things, doing groceries, cleaning up after the kids, having the energy to carry out all my usual household chores and tasks."

Coach: "It sounds like you have a lot on your hands currently, how much time could you commit to exercise?"

Client: "Well, I want to commit to exercise as much as possible, every day!"

Coach: "I love your enthusiasm! Have you tried exercise or lifestyle improvements before?"

Client: "Yes, I have tried some booty band workouts on Instagram but lost motivation after a week."

Coach: "Do you believe that exercise every day would be an achievable and realistic goal for you right now?"

Client: "I would like to think so ..."

Coach: "What potential barriers could you see arising that may get in the way of you exercising every day?"

Client: "Time, kids, family, energy levels, motivation."

Coach: Ok, well, how about we keep things simple for the time being? I suggest a more conservative approach, get some small wins under your belt and then we can always add more movement as you progress and develop a sustainable routine that fits your lifestyle!"

Client: "But I want to achieve my goal as quickly as possible."

Coach: "Maintaining your health is a life-long pursuit, rather than striving for a fixed point, view it as a continuous thing if you want to put these habits in place for life. So, it's best to start simple and make sustainable steps in creating the life you want."

Client: "You know what, that actually sounds a lot better."

Coach: "Great! So, we know you want to lose weight. Now let's get a bit more specific, how much and by when?"

Client: "I would like to lose 5kg and increase the definition in the back of my arms by, say, September this year."

Coach: "That is definitely an achievable goal within the next four months. What are you not willing to do to achieve this goal?"

Client: "Not willing to do? Hmm, I don't want to bust myself doing cardio every day, I prefer weights. I don't want to have to give up the things I love like socialising just because I'm on a diet."

Coach: "That is perfectly fine! We can definitely work around events and find the style of exercise you prefer. There will be commitments you must make though, like sticking to your programme, adhering to the lifestyle advice that's suited for you and staying consistent overall."

People make goals every day. Some are good, some not so good. Just like the variables of good programmes we spoke about previously, there are certain factors we want to account for and crack down on to give us a well-rounded goal.

First, what is a goal?

"Goals are the road maps that guide you to your destination." – Roy T. Bennett

Have you ever heard of SMART goals?

This is a simple concept to give you a framework for your initial attempts at goal setting.

SMART stands for Specific, Measurable, Attainable, Realistic, Timely.

Let's look at each of those qualities in detail:

SPECIFIC

Now, in the above scenario, we can see that this woman was specific about her goal of losing 5kg and improving the definition of the back of her arms by September.

Being specific is essential with any goal to allow us to build our programming around this.

If someone came to you with the goal of running a marathon and yet all you gave them for their programme was handstands, it's pretty obvious we won't get a good result with this person. Similarly, if another person came to you with a vague goal, replying "I don't know" when asked why they walked in that day, then we have no clear objective. This, again, makes it very difficult.

Having a clear, identified goal is your first step, a starting point. That will give you direction and purpose.

Once the goal is determined we must look at the other variables.

MEASURABLE

So, you want to achieve the goal that you have identified. How do we measure this?

Some ideas related to health and fitness could be regular body weight girth measurements, photos, body weight on the scales and so on.

If it's a goal outside of the health industry, such as being a better friend to somebody, how do we measure this?

In this instance, we might measure how well we listen to our friends. Next question, how do we measure how well we listen? Through time. We may use the metric of how many minutes we spend talking to them on the phone each week. For example, an acquaintance may be a few minutes a week, a good friend may be 20-30 minutes per week. Other areas you can measure may include: how supportive we are, how much time we spend with one another communicating across the day, week, month.

If we do not measure, how do we know if we have achieved our goal or are at least moving in the direction of achieving it?

Get clear on this. It is of utmost importance.

ATTAINABLE

You come to me with the goal of speaking fluent Spanish by Tuesday next week, yet you've never taken a Spanish lesson in your life.

This is a specific goal, we can measure it by the simple fact of your speaking Spanish fluently or not, but is this attainable?

Unless you are a secret linguistical genius, I'm going to have to say good luck, but no chance.

Goals must be attainable; are you trying to achieve too much in a short amount of time?

Think back to our scenario of a bad programme – doing too much, too soon. As humans we have limits, as much as some of us would like to think otherwise.

Everyone has a biological limit. We can't grow wings and fly spontaneously, although it would be pretty awesome.

We can't be a professional at something just because we have the thought to be; rather, we must be diligent and practice, often over extended periods of time.

For a goal to be attainable, ensure you have the right process in place – enough time, an action plan and something to keep you accountable.

REALISTIC

I want to bench press a truck vs. I want to bench press 100kg.

What is more realistic?

I'm going to go out on a limb and assume you aren't the incredible hulk, so only the latter may still be within your reach.

Having a goal that is realistic goes hand in hand with it being attainable. Our goals need to be based in reality or the reality will be that we fail.

A more subtle issue that can arise when we set goals is not knowing enough information about the goal in the first place. That may include what is actually required to achieve said goal.

Do you know off the top of your head how much weight is appropriate to lose when aiming to revamp your body composition to lose weight?

Or, put another way, how much weight is reasonable and sustainable to lose per week and how long should you even spend dieting?

Well, the answers are approximately 1% of body weight per week, e.g., if you're 100kg then 1kg per week, and roughly eight to 12 weeks is the sweet spot for dieting, as too long can lead to increased stress psychologically and physically.

Before knowing this, you may only have a show like *The Biggest Loser* as a reference point for weight loss. They can lose 10-20kg in some weeks, which is insane! You might be thinking, *I should be able to lose that 5kg in no time at all!*

This sets us up for unrealistic expectations and goals from the get-go.

TIME-BASED

Each element of a SMART goal adds a layer to the preceding one.

Time is an objective component that holds us accountable. Time-based goals create urgency, giving us a predetermined moment where we will know whether we have achieved or failed to reach our goal. We can use the time to create multiple goals, both in the long and short term.

I'd suggest short-term goals are under six months; long-term goals exceed six months.

EXAMPLE

"It is now January and my new year's resolution is to lose 10kg of fat mass by December of this year (within 12 months)."

This is a long-term goal, it ticks a few of our boxes. It's specific, we can measure it and it's realistic.

Now that we have a clear objective for the future, we can develop an action plan or a short-term plan to enable us to reach this end goal. Enter ... the short-term goals.

Breaking down our long-term goal into bite-sized chunks is one of the ways we can ensure we are meeting our goal step by step. Creating short-term targets to help you reach your long-term goal is an effective way to ensure it is measured, attainable and realistic to achieve by a certain date. Your short-term goals may, for example, to be to lose a fraction of the weight you plan to lose overall within a certain timeframe. This does not need to be linear.

For example, losing approximately 0.25kg per week, which equals 1kg a month. After 10 months you would have achieved your goal in a perfect world where nothing goes wrong.

So, was this specific? Yep, Was this measured? Yep, Attainable and realistic? Yep, Time based? Yep!

Great, we just completed a SMART goal. How easy was that?!

If I'm being honest, this above goal is very superficial. It ticks the boxes of a SMART goal, but it doesn't really tell us how we are going to do this, the barriers in our way or why we are doing it in the first place.

Let's apply this to another goal. You and I want to build a house by the end of the year. Cool, we can definitely do it, but we haven't figured out how, what roadblocks may come up and why we want this house to be built. The action behind our goal is missing, so even with all of the elements of the SMART acronym checked we can fail.

SMART goals can only take us so far. It is simply a tool, so don't get bogged down and consumed by it. There is research that suggests SMART goals aren't even based on evidence, they lack guidance, have redundant criteria and often aren't used correc tly.[41] Yes, I know I just wrote a spiel about why you should use SMART goals! I'm not here to reinvent the wheel, just to make it better!

I would revamp the model to incorporate a foolproof goal. One jam-packed with potential barriers you may come across, a clear-ly defined 'why' and a methodology to achieve our goal, espe-cially when things get saucy and roadblocks pop up to distract or deter us. Unfortunately, SMART goals alone don't currently do this.

Barriers to our goals

An often-overlooked concept is the barriers we will face once our goal is set. Do you want to build a house?

Barriers with this example may include:

- Finances

- Government restrictions

- Designs

- Location

- Timing

- Availability of materials

Take a moment to work on your own goal, preferably something long-term (more than six months).

Use the above concepts to start formulating a specific, measurable and achievable goal for yourself. Next, try and break down this goal into smaller short-term goals, and figure out how you will measure if you are moving towards, staying still or moving away from your long-term goal.

Now is the time to delve into a few more concepts.

If we go back to the person wanting to lose weight, what are some potential barriers that you can envision preventing success?

SOME AREAS THAT COME TO MIND FOR ME ARE:

- Being surrounded by family and friends that mock you for trying to lose weight.

- Having a lack of time due to family commitments.

- Not knowing how to lose weight or lacking the resources to meet your desires.

Barriers suck. However, the silver lining is that planning for these barriers can prevent a lot of headaches down the track.

Now, I know what you're thinking: I'm not a fortune teller. You're right, you aren't. I don't expect you to have a crystal ball that tells you every possible scenario, but you need to be aware that you will face obstacles irrespective of what your end goal may be.

What I want you to take away from this is the importance of planning. Have a rough guide of the large barriers you may face, even if this is purely at a face value, and then write down how you would overcome them.

This concept is based on Tim Ferriss' "fear setting" exercises.

Fear setting is a helpful way of identifying the worst things that can happen to you. This allows you to come up with solutions for minimising or overcoming these disastrous barriers and then repairing any damage caused.

Now, I am not going to try and explain it better than Tim, so go and watch his Ted Talk – "Why you should identify your fears instead of your goals."

You're back? Cool, so we are on the same page now.

WHY

Ever since coming across this concept, I have become somewhat obsessed.

Your 'why' is the reason you get out of bed, the reason you want to train, and the reason you started reading this book in the first place. Each decision we make has a 'why' behind it, conscious or subconscious, and we are guided and dictated to by our whys.

Have you ever questioned the motive or driving force behind the decisions you make?

Throughout my life, I have often pondered on, questioned and reflected upon the notion of 'why'.

If I feel myself start to waver in confidence, happiness, passion or ambition I will ask myself why. What events or series of events are occurring? What am I not doing to fulfil these areas in my life?

Why am I writing this book? Well, I want to help you. But why? I have developed the belief that I have a purpose which intertwines with my life. My purpose is to help; I want to spread a message of empowerment through my own knowledge and experiences to enable people to become the best versions of themselves. I will constantly ask myself why this is, and I have thought up reasons such as my environment, my upbringing, the books I've read or the conversations I've had. Maybe I am the summation of all of these; maybe there's something deeper than all of this, driving me to my 'why' of helping you and everyone I can.

Let me take you into my mind for a moment, back to when I was a wee lad, playing soccer at roughly five years old. I looked up at the sky, it looked back at me. Cloudy, angry, as if it was ready to explode and drench the terrain I was standing on. I looked to the freshly-mown hills in the distance to see if my parents were watching me from above. The game had just kicked off, the ball was getting kicked around left, right and centre. Kids were running around like puppies chasing a tennis ball. I was the same, rushing in, my goal to chase and get the ball by any means. A kid in just front of me now had the ball, and I saw my chance. I lunged forward, and the kid slides the ball out of the way like a magician using sleight of hand (ok, maybe a novice magician as this kid forgot to move his leg as well). While he was performing magic, I was still mid-lunge. Instead of the ball, I found his leg with the stud of my weathered soccer boots as I came crashing down. The kid fell to the ground, and the game carried on. I stopped in my tracks. My goal was not the ball anymore, I forgot about the game altogether. Instead, my aim was to help this person. Undo my wrong and make sure he was ok. I reached out my hand and I helped him to his feet as the rest of the puppies frantically chased the ball.

This is a moment I keep coming back to in my thoughts. The first time, I remember being selfless and helping someone because I could. I was elated, I had a moment of pure satisfaction; this is an aspect of my character I am still proud of to this day. Call it child-like innocence or remorse, but in that moment, I felt a spark, the gift of helping others. From that moment I knew that whatever I did with my life, it had to revolve around helping people. People like you.

So, here I am today. Reflecting on my why while writing about how you can find yours. Look to your memories, the moments you remember before the cruelty, the social pressures and the failed dreams made you become who you are today. Unravel yourself, peeling away all of the expectations, things you've told yourself and things you've read to get to your essence. The core of you.

Throughout my life, I have learnt many things and unlearnt probably just as much. Please now take a moment to reflect. Try to figure out the why behind what you do; you may not have the answer today. That's ok. Stay with it though, come back to it throughout your life. Figure out your why and let it guide you to help you achieve what you are meant to.

WHAT ARE THE BENEFITS OF GOAL SETTING?

Throughout this chapter, you have learned about the intricacies, problems and difficulties we may face with goal setting. It seems like a lot of work to clearly define our goals, identify roadblocks and take actionable steps towards achieving what we have set for ourselves.

Do you know what I'm going to ask next?

'Why' are we doing this?

Goal setting is a powerful tool which can have a beneficial impact throughout our entire lives. It can be the catalyst for behavioural change, learning new skills, undoing trauma and bettering yourself. Goal setting can be the tool to align your focus, adding fuel to your ambition and igniting change.

The goals we set for ourselves become a part of us

You have a choice about who and what you want to become through using this tool. Use goal setting wisely and reap the benefits throughout your life.

The psychology around goal setting is huge! Let's get technical for a little bit.

There are multiple psychology models around decision-making. I prefer the transtheoretical model when looking at people throughout the stages of change. The transtheoretical model places people into categories for their readiness to change.[42]

1. Precontemplation

2. Contemplation

3. Preparation

4. Action

5. Maintenance

PRECONTEMPLATION

This is the initial stage. The thought hasn't even entered the person's consciousness yet. They are unassuming and unchanging in their thoughts, behaviours and actions. Imagine Mr Bean; ignorance is bliss, right? This stage is often ignited when someone makes you aware of a fault, behaviour or skill that you aren't adept in.

CONTEMPLATION

The conscious mind is now aware of a variable that can be changed. This may be a specific behaviour such as wanting to give up smoking or wanting to learn how to perform a dance move/routine.

PREPARATION

This person is now seeking guidance on how to make a change; they are reading, learning, and asking for help regarding the behaviour they wish to change.

This is a vital stage – this may be where you start to set your goals and work out the pathway to achieving your chosen behavioural change. Do not skip this step; there is a strong correlation between skipping this step and failing to achieve a behavioural change.

Remember what I said earlier: "Fail to prepare, prepare to fail."

ACTION

This person is now equipped: they have prepared (hopefully) to make a meaningful change in behaviour, whether it's a new behaviour or cessation of poor behaviour. This is where the execution of the plan from the preparation phase is carried out.

MAINTENANCE

Can you guess what I'm about to say? Maintenance is another vital stage, hell, they all are. This is where we continue our new behaviour. We aim to carry out and maintain our new-formed behaviour as part of us moving forward.

WAIT, HOW DO WE ACHIEVE OUR GOAL?

While our goal is essential, I would argue the process that enables our goal to be achieved is more important. The goal is our direction, our endpoint if you will. The question remains, how do we reach the endpoint?

Without creating actionable steps to achieve our said goal, we are lost. Consider what separates success from failure, winning from losing, first from last. Each person sets out with goals, often the same one e.g., to win!

What separates them in this is the actionable steps they take to get them there, the processes they create and embody to achieve their task.

If I had a goal to lose weight like our above example at the start of this chapter, I can do one of the following: either adhere to my nutrition advice and hit my calorie targets, train regularly, get adequate sleep to recover, mitigate barriers that may deter me from completing the above tasks; on the other hand, I can set my goal of weight loss and miss some sessions, binge eat here and there at social gatherings, not track what I'm eating and then question why I haven't achieved my goal. The actionable steps we take are key.

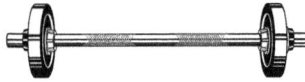

Putting it all together

We've covered a lot so far, so I've summarised the main concepts below for ease of reference.

Step 1 – Setting a goal

You set a goal of wanting to become a respected and knowledgeable coach by the end of the year.

Step 2 – Understanding your why

You want to do this because you have a deep desire to help as many people as you can, you are passionate about health and fitness and want to give people the highest quality service you can by constantly re-evaluating and improving your service.

Step 3 – Identifying and overcoming your barriers

You've noticed that a lack of knowledge and experience is blocking your path, so you seek educational resources like books and courses to further your knowledge, skills and expertise.

Step 4 – Creating your action plan using the transtheoretical model

For this step, it will be useful to understand where you are in your readiness to complete your goal. In the following example, we will imagine you are a coach.

At one point you were in the pre-contemplation stage, when you didn't know about a lack of knowledge in a particular area of health or care about it until possibly a client came to you with a question or a problem you didn't know how to address. This leads to the urge to get better.

You are now in the contemplation stage, a place where you are conscious of needing to upskill your health knowledge and skills, you have been dealing with a client who isn't getting results and you don't have the answers.

Enter the preparation stage: you know that you want to upskill and become a respected and knowledgeable coach, so how do you get there? You start doing some research into reputable courses and books that may help you upskill, even looking at potential mentors to guide you through your journey. During this stage you map out that you will actively engage in reading 20-30 pages per night for the next couple of months, you will also engage with a respected online mentoring service for two to four hours per week to enable you to improve your knowledge, test your skills and increase awareness on areas you may be lacking.

You are now in the action stage. You have purchased a number of educational textbooks/studies, you are enrolled in a course with a mentor and you now decide to move towards your goal of improving your knowledge by actively partaking in all the activities set for you. The action stage is where we will make or break our goal. Without engaging with our well-laid plans from the preparation phase by reading books about health and fitness or upskilling through educational courses, how can we expect to achieve success?

The final stage is maintenance. We have read the books and completed the course. Now what? We have the answer to our previous client's questions and feel we are a much better coach than we were when we set our goal at the start of the year.

Are we done? NO.

Information is constantly changing, and we will never have all the answers, and the endeavour to be a knowledgeable and wise person should be a lifelong journey. This is often what separates some people from others. We have actionable steps that we must perform to reach our goal, but then what? If we stop there we may go backwards, fall out of touch with the latest knowledge and lose respect for failing to keep up with current trends, information and best practice.

In order to maintain our status, we must build upon our existing knowledge and continue to work towards the goal of becoming a better trainer. You will need to pick up another book, listen to another podcast or another course and so on. Being up to date with ever-changing research and its practical implications is, in essence, the maintenance of your goal.

If you follow this step-by-step approach, how can you not reach success in whatever field you choose?

As I said earlier, this process may not be linear. Maybe you get to the preparation stage and figure out you're not passionate about finding the answer and instead wish to shift your focus somewhere else. Maybe you don't reach the next phase because life gets in the way or you failed to complete your actionable steps to the degree required.

Understanding the intricacies and actionable steps of goal setting, and the psychology that people go through when setting and moving through their goals, is essential for all of us if we are to reach the desired outcomes.

For me, this was a game changer. It assisted in me actually reaching the goals I set in all areas of my life – business, relationships, self-development – and ultimately shaped who I am as a person. This is powerful stuff, and when used correctly can propel you forward in life.

Life isn't all sunshine and rainbows

It is worth mentioning the other side of the coin. The actionable steps we take can be determinantal, just as much as they can be beneficial. The steps we take to achieve our goals create habits, and if we consistently miss our actionable steps, we create stronger connections to this path.

We are all wired differently.

No doubt you have experienced this and have certain predispositions in certain areas of your life, areas where you struggle to excel or commonly find yourself procrastinating.

We need to show compassion and empathy when setting goals for ourselves. If we attack ourselves or set expectations that are unachievable, we will fall into old patterns. Instead, we must look to undertake actionable steps, identify barriers that blocked our way and find a way to overcome them in order to take new, positive strides towards a healthier lifestyle.

13

Back to Basics

"You've baked a really lovely cake, but then you've used dog shit for frosting." - Steve Jobs

We are finally at the point of action; how to structure and implement training programmes, where to start, formats and more. This chapter should leave you with templates you can adapt, the understanding of why you are using them and the ability to get creative in how you plan your own programmes. These programmes will be specifically designed around gym-based movements, but you can certainly apply the concepts and styles to other areas (yes, I will give insight into how as well).

We have covered goal setting, training principles, methodologies and periodisation. This is where we combine the four approaches to make effective programmes, enabling you to achieve your goals.

Where do we start?

Well, like a number of concepts I've covered, why not start with the end?

Long-term goal setting is a surefire way to success. Understand what your end goal looks like, and then break it down into bite-sized chunks: daily and weekly habits that enable us to get there. I want you to keep a holistic outlook. View each programme you use as a piece in the puzzle of your success. What are your goals? Do they need updating? What's your level of ability, injury history, time constraints, lifestyle and how are the stressors in your life at the moment?

These formats will be generic rather than specific to an archetype so I can show you my thought process. You can add your own flavour as you see fit. I will now take you through my method of thinking when creating long-term programmes; where I start and the rationale behind it.

Each programme will be four weeks unless I specify otherwise. Each programme will involve between one and four programmed days depending on what is needed. For this generic programme, I will start, well, at the beginning, contrary to what I said before, so you can see a sequential flow to the patterning and progression.

LANGUAGE

To ensure I'm ticking the box of communicating well, I want you to understand the language and terminology I will be referring to. If you get lost, refer back to the list below to get a quick snapshot of what the hell I'm talking about.

Term:	Definition:	Term:	Definition:
Horizontal Push / Pull	Any movement that works perpendicular or across from gravity (left and right). Think of seated rows or face pulls and bench presses or push ups.	RPE	Rate of perceived exertion – how difficult the exercise is on a modified scale of one to 10. One is easy, 10 is extremely difficult.
Vertical Push / Pull	Any movement that works in parallel with gravity (up and down). Think of movements like shoulder presses and lat pulldowns or chin ups.	RIR	Repetitions in reserve. This refers to how many repetitions the individual is away from failure of an exercise.
Knee Dominant	Any motion pertaining to the articulation of the pelvis, knee and ankles. Movements include squatting, lunging, split squats, step ups, vertical jumping.	Co-contraction	The simultaneous ability of muscles to contract to stabilise a joint. Common examples are the calf and hamstrings to stabilise the knee joint or the bicep and forearms to stabilise the elbow joint.
Hinge Dominant	Any motion pertaining to articulation of the pelvis – deadlifts, kettlebell swings, glute bridges, broad jumps are common exercises within this category.	Super Sets	Two exercises paired together before a rest.
Core	The interplay between all the muscles and tendons from the trunk down to the thighs. They work in three dimensions –all planes of motion. Think leg raises, planking, side planking.	Tri-Sets	Three exercises paired together before a rest.
		Giant Sets	Four exercises paired together before a rest.
Accessory	Any motions that are smaller and more focused on the internal muscles that can assist the prime movers to complete their role. E.g., the rotator cuff assisting the deltoid to move the shoulder. Movements include: farmer's carry, bicep curls and triceps extensions.	Circuit	Five exercises paired together before a rest.
		Sets	The amount of time you will complete a number of repetitions.
		Reps	The amount of repetitions or repeats of an exercise.

Figure 13.1

Term:	Definition:
Tempo	How fast you engage with the exercise 1st # = eccentric portion. 2nd #= pause at the bottom of the movement. 3rd #=- concentric portion. 4th #= pause at the top of the movement.
Underhand Grip (UH)	Any motion that your palm faces upwards (towards the roof).
Overhand Grip (OH)	Any motion that your palm faces downwards (towards the floor).
Single Limb (SL)	The use of only one limb during the exercise. E.g., bent over dumbbell row or alternating lunges.
As Many Rounds as Possible (AMRAP)	This refers to a circuit format. You set an arbitrary time limit and perform as many rounds as you can.
Metabolic	This refers to a style of training focused on bouts of intense weighted effort followed by rest intervals. E.g. Squat Jumping for 30s then KB swings for 30s followed by a short rest and repeat.
Cardio Interval	This is defined as high intenstiy cardiovascular movements (rhythmic nature) such as running, swimming or cycling. Perform these for time bouts like 30s on, 30s off.
Carry	A carry is one of the primal movement patterns discussed earlier. This can be any variation of holding weight e.g. farmers carry, zercher carry, single arm (SA) carry.

Figure 13.2

PROGRAM I: 0-4 WEEKS

GIANT SETS FOR ONE-WEEK CLIENT

Exercise	Sets	Reps	Rest	Tempo
A1. Horizontal Push A2. Knee Dominant A3. Horizontal Pull A4. Hinge Dominant	2	20R	60s	3010
B1. Core B2. Loaded Carry B3. Accessory Lower B4. Accessory Upper	2	20R	60s	3010

Figure 13.3

GIANT SETS FOR TWO-WEEK CLIENT

Day 1				
Exercise	Sets	Reps	Rest	Tempo
A1. Horizontal Push A2. Unilateral Squat A3. Horizontal Pull A4. Unilateral Hinge	2	20R	60s	3010
B1. Core B2. Loaded Carry B3. Accessory Lower B4. Accessory Upper	3	10-12R	60s	3010
Day 2				
Exercise	Sets	Reps	Rest	Tempo
A1. Bilateral Hinge A2. Vertical Push A3. Bilateral Squat A4. Vertical Pull	2	20R	60s	3010
B1. Core B2. Lower Co-Contraction B3. Upper Co-Contraction B4. Metabolic / Cardio	3	10-12R	60s	3010

Figure 13.4

Rationale

This programme involves low sets with high repetitions. Why? you ask.

Well, I want to elicit adaptation. We know from research that novices require relatively little stimulus to create the environment for adaptation. We also know from the stages of learning that we will require high frequency to improve upon the skill or movement patterns that we are training.

Within this programme, I am not too concerned with leaning towards muscle or fat loss, rather the aim is to educate the individual on skill acquisition, quality of movement and understanding basic movement principles and patterns. Research shows that within a newbie programme we can get simultaneous muscle growth and fat loss. In my opinion, focusing too much on one approach is wasted at this stage. To create more resilient and versatile human beings, start with a solid base and it will be much easier to add later. If we fail to establish this base, our training endeavours may not last long as injuries, chronic tightness and pain may start to creep in.

PROGRAM 2: 5-8 WEEKS
ALTERNATING SUPERSETS FOR TWICE PER WEEK

Day 1				
Exercise	Sets	Reps	Rest	Tempo
A1. Vertical Push A2. Hinge Dominant	3	10-15R	60s	3010
B1. Vertical Pull B2. Knee Dominant	3	10-15R	60s	3010
C1. SA Carry C2. Lower Accessory C3. Upper Accessory	3	15-20R	60s	3010
Day 2				
Exercise	Sets	Reps	Rest	Tempo
A1. Horizontal Pull A2. SL Knee Dominant	3	10-15R	60s	3010
B1. Horizontal Push B2. SL Hip Dominant	3	10-15R	60s	3010
C1. Core - Transverse C2. Lower Accessory C3. Upper Accessory	3	15-20R	60s	3010

Figure 13.5

RATIONALE

We have progressed from giant sets to super sets. The main factor that we want to change is intensity. Now that the novice has completed their first programme, we want to keep similar movement patterns while creating a greater stimulus.

The intensity of this format (5-8 weeks) will elicit a greater stimulus in the individual simply by moving from giant sets to super sets. This is due to our variable of rest: within a giant set you may complete the first exercise, then the second through to the fourth before having your rest period. Contrast this with our second programme which sees us perform super sets, in which we immediately increase the intensity of our exercise by having a smaller rest period, essentially half of the two to three minutes you get with giant sets.

Our participant is still learning the cognitive stage of skill acquisition. Repeated exposure through 10-15R will encourage continued adaptation through their training phases.

PROGRAM 3: 9-12 WEEKS

ANTAGONIST SUPERSETS + ACCESSORY

Day 1				
Exercise	Sets	Reps	Rest	Tempo
A1. Vertical Push A2. Vertical Pull	4	10-12R	90s	3010
B1. Horziontal Push B2. Horizontal Pull	4	10-12R	90s	3010
C1. Unilateral Knee Dominant C2. Unilateral Hinge Dominant C3. Lower Co-Contraction C4. Hip Accessory	3	12-15R	60s	3010
Day 2				
Exercise	Sets	Reps	Rest	Tempo
A1. Vertical Knee Dominant A2. Vertical Hip Dominant	4	10-12R	90s	3010
B1. Horziontal Knee Dominant B2. Jump Variation	4	10-12R	90s	3010
C1. Unilateral Push C2. Unilateral Pull C3. Elbow Extension C4. Elbow Flexion	3	12-15R	60s	3010

Figure 13.6

RATIONAL

The key change here is to the order of exercises, shifting to super sets to encourage greater adaptation. We have now split our sessions, still using the whole body but placing greater emphasis on our first two series, the A and B series of super sets. Day 1 involves an emphasis on the upper body, with Day 2 focusing on the lower body. The title of antagonist super sets refers to the combining of opposite actions – push and pull, for example. This is one way to allow the body to perform an exercise and work a separate area, for example:

Pushing involves the triceps, shoulders, and pectoral musculature.

Pulling involves the biceps, shoulders, latissimus dorsi and rhomboid musculature.

There is some transfer in fatigue, however, the primary areas working will get a much-needed rest while you train opposing areas. Win, win.

The accessories in the C-series are opposing, with Day 1 focusing on the lower body and Day 2 on the upper body. This allows greater emphasis all round: generally, what we do first is what we do best. By separating the upper and lower body components we are still essentially 'fresh' for our accessory movements. In my experience, these are notorious for a participant being lacklustre; low energy and effort is applied towards the end of the workout due to the accumulation of peripheral fatigue from the earlier exercises. We can mitigate this with the format of our programme, which revitalises the accessory movements by ensuring we carry them out with the same intensity and focus as our main movements.

PROGRAM 4: 13-16 WEEKS HYPERTROPHY

Day 1				
Exercise	Sets	Reps	Rest	Tempo
A1. Vertical Push A2. Hinge Dominant	4	10-15R	90s	3010
B1. Vertical Pull B2. Knee Dominant	4	10-15R	90s	3010
C1. SA Carry C2. Lower Accessory C3. Upper Accessory	3	15-20R	60s	3010
Day 2				
Exercise	Sets	Reps	Rest	Tempo
A1. Horizontal Pull A2. SL Knee Dominant	4	10-15R	90s	3010
B1. Horizontal Push B2. SL Hip Dominant	4	10-15R	90s	3010
C1. Core - Transverse C2. Lower Accessory C3. Upper Accessory	3	15-20R	60s	3010

Figure 13.7

FAT LOSS

Day 1				
Exercise	Sets	Reps	Rest	Tempo
A1. Vertical Push A2. Hinge Dominant A3. Vertical Pull A4. Bilateral Squat A5. Metabolic A6. Cardio Interval	3	10-15R	120s	3010
Day 2				
Exercise	Sets	Reps	Rest	Tempo
A1. Horizontal Pull A2. SL Knee Dominant A3. Horizontal Push A4. Carry A5. Metabolic A6. Core	3	10-15R	120s	3010

Figure 13.8

RATIONALE

After roughly three months of training, this is where I will branch out and dial down on the specifics of a person's goal. This is not the case for everyone and must be adapted, especially if they come to you with time-specific goals; but for the large majority, we need to take the time to create healthy patterns of movement.

This entails allowing time for the individual to progress through the stages of learning to understand and develop proprioception within their bodies to ensure movement proficiency can be maintained. This should occur before we start implementing advanced training techniques. Think of this like a video game in which you have to acquire certain skills and weapons before you can take on the boss at the end of each level. To give you an idea of how this might apply to different goals, I have created two streams.

One is more focused towards a healthy individual in the general population that wishes to grow muscle (hypertrophy), and the other is for someone who wishes to improve body composition through fat loss. As you can see from the two streams, the key difference in our hypertrophy and fat loss programmes lies within in the formatting. The exercises or movement patterns will be largely the same, but the structure of how we perform these will alter.

Within the fat loss programme, we are looking to expend a lot of energy. A versatile and effective way to do this is to alternate multi-joint, multi-muscle movement patterns between the upper and lower body, which requires high oxygen and metabolic demand. In contrast, within our hypertrophy programme we will look to accrue metabolic fatigue and time under tension through a combination of volume and high relative intensity (>70% of our one rep maximum).

PROGRAM 5: 17-20 WEEKS

HYPERTROPHY

Day 1				
Exercise	Sets	Reps	Rest	Tempo
A1. Vertical Pull A2. Vertical Push	4	10-15R	90s	3010
B1. SL Vertical Pull B2. SL Vertical Push	4	10-15R	90s	3010
C1. SA Carry C2. Elbow Flexion C3. Elbow Extension	3	15-20R	60s	3010
Day 2				
Exercise	Sets	Reps	Rest	Tempo
A1. Knee Dominant A2. Hip Dominant	4	10-15R	90s	3010
B1. SL Knee Dominant B2. SL Hip Dominant	4	10-15R	90s	3010
C1. Core - Transverse C2. Lower Accessory C3. Lower Co-contraction	3	15-20R	60s	3010

Figure 13.9

Fat Loss

Day 1				
Exercise	Sets	Reps	Rest	Tempo
A1. Vertical Push A2. Hip Dominant A3. Vertical Pull A4. Bilateral Squat A5. Metabolic A6. Cardio Interval	4	10-15R	120s	3010
Finisher AMRAP: B1. Body Weight Knee Dominant B2. Body Weight Horizontal Push	1	10m	NA	As required
Day 2				
Exercise	Sets	Reps	Rest	Tempo
A1. Horizontal Pull A2. SL Knee Dominant A3. Horizontal Push A4. Carry A5. Metabolic A6. Core	4	10-15R	120s	3010
Finisher AMRAP: B1. Body Weight Hip Dominant B2. Body Weight Horizontal Pull	1	10m	NA	As required

Figure 13.10

Rationale

Here, we continue to branch out into hypertrophy and fat loss. Both body composition programmes utilise similar repetitions and set schemes, the difference again lies in the formatting. By now it must be becoming evident just how creative you can be with your format.

We have utilised super sets and varying rest intervals, as well as splitting our programme into upper and lower body days. The fat loss programme continues with a full-body approach but with a circuit style.

Within this stage and the next, you can add finishers. A finisher refers to a small, high-intensity block to stimulate further calorie expenditure, particularly useful for our fat loss protocols. This finisher may come in the form of 'every minute on the minute' or EMOM, 'as many rounds as possible' (AMRAP) or a host of other methods to elicit high volume and intensity in a short time period.

Program 6: 21-24 Weeks

Hypertrophy

Day 1				
Exercise	Sets	Reps	Rest	Tempo
A1. Vertical Pull A2. Vertical Push	4	8-10R	90s	3010
B1. SL Vertical Pull B2. SL Vertical Push	4	8-10R	90s	3010
C1. SA Carry C2. Elbow Flexion C3. Elbow Extension	3	10-12R	60s	3010
Day 2				
Exercise	Sets	Reps	Rest	Tempo
A1. Knee Dominant A2. Hip Dominant	4	8-10R	60s	3010
B1. SL Knee Dominant B2. SL Hip Dominant	4	8-10R	60s	3010
C1. Core - Transverse C2. Lower Accessory C3. Lower Co-contraction	3	10-12R	60s	3010

Figure 13.11

Fat Loss

Day 1				
Exercise	Sets	Reps	Rest	Tempo
A1. Vertical Push A2. Hip Dominant A3. Vertical Pull A4. Cardio Interval	4	10-15R	120s	3010
B1. Knee Dominant B2. Vertical Pull B3. Carry B4. Metabolic Interval	4	10-15R	120s	As required
Day 1				
Exercise	Sets	Reps	Rest	Tempo
A1. Horizontal Push A2. Hip Dominant A3. Horizontal Pull A4. Cardio Interval	4	10-15R	120s	3010
B1. SL Knee Dominant B2. Core B3. Carry B4. Metabolic Interval	4	10-15R	120s	As required

Figure 13.12

RATIONALE

We are now close to moving someone into the intermediate stage of training. If you worked through the previous programmes, you should now be capable of utilising your body within the primal movement patterns of squatting, hinging, pushing, pulling and carrying. You'll likely even have a grasp of your relative rate of perceived exertions and can modify the intensity to get your desired outcome.

This programme further narrows down the specific training for hypertrophy and fat loss. For hypertrophy, we are looking to target specific muscles to elicit growth through our super sets and overloading methods. For fat loss, we are looking at the entire body expending a lot of energy through multiple circuits / giant sets.

LINEAR PROGRESSION VS. UNDULATING PROGRESSION

It is worth mentioning the two main styles of rep schemes, linear and undulating, which you can use to vary your programme.

Linear progression refers to sequential descension or ascension in our periodisation scheme. In layman's terms, we go from highest to lowest or lowest to highest. This may come in the form of repetitions: in programme one we do 20 repetitions for a particular exercise, in programme two we do 15 repetitions, programme three may involve 8-12 repetitions and so on.

With undulating, however, there is no clear progression. An example of this may be performing 15 repetitions within programme one, then eight repetitions in programme two, before going to 12-15 repetitions in programme three.

At the time of writing in 2022, experts are divided on whether one works better than the other. This is where we need to tailor our schemes for the person: their goals, history, wants and needs. These different repetition schemes can be a useful tool to adjust the degrees of challenge to the individual. Personally, I use a combination of both repetition styles. Typically, I will start with a linear progression, as evident throughout the six programmes I wrote above, before progressing to an undulating method as the trainee becomes more advanced.

At the end of the day, our bodies cannot count repetitions. The overload principles work on progressive overload that is stimulated primarily through time under tension and metabolite accrual. This means that as long as you are using muscles frequently and with a decent intensity – think seven to eight RPE – you will be fine. This is all about personal preference and, again, context matters, so tailor the needs to the individual or team.

CARDIOVASCULAR TRAINING

We know from our physical activity guidelines that we require resistance-based training utilising the style of training above for our bones, nerves, tendons and muscular systems. These guidelines indicate we need cardiovascular (cardio) training for our heart, arteriole and venous systems. Rather than give you a month-by-month breakdown, I will detail some methods you may wish to utilise for light-moderate and high-intensity cardio training. Firstly, what movements classify as cardio?

Think of movements with a cyclical or rhythmical nature. This pertains to running, walking, cycling, jumping even weight-based circuits. Any physical activity that elevates your heart rate and sustains this for some time. Cardio training and development of the energy systems will rely on your understanding of your heart rate and the intensity zones.

To find your maximum heart rate (HR) use the following equation.

'220 - 'your age"

Example: 30-year-old

220 – 30 = 190 beats per minute (bpm)

That's it. Now everything else will be a percentage of your maximum HR. What are the intensities again?

Low – Moderate = 50-85% max HR

High / Vigorous = 85-100% max HR

Now we know what it is, do you remember the energy system archetypes we spoke about in Chapter 7?

We had three distinct archetypes for energy usage which will dictate our training.

Utilisation limitation = Muscle

Delivery limitation = Heart

Respiration limitation = Lungs

UTILISATION LIMITATION

For our utilisation limitation subgroup, start with the above training programs to develop the necessary muscle, and then you can transition into delivery and respiration style training based on your requirements. I would suggest you focus on low-moderate intensity-based cardio training through some of the below methods.

- **Low-intensity steady state (LISS)** – This means keeping your heart rate within the desired intensity range for a continuous effort.

- **Intervals** – Build your aerobic capacity by alternating between higher and lower intensities. An example may be to walk 100m or 30s then run 100m or 30s for the desired range of period e.g. 2km or 20 minutes.

DELIVERY LIMITATION

These are the people that are generally muscle-bound. They have spent a decent time within a gym or sports setting gaining muscle. The goal for this archetype is to desaturate (decrease oxygen in the blood) but not exhaust this completely. How do we know if we are completely desaturated? Well, we will get a pump. Generally, our delivery-limited people will start cycling, for example, they will eventually fatigue due to the burning sensation or 'pump' within the legs rather than due to shortness of breath. The work for this is in the style of training.

- **Interval-based training** – Focusing on low tension and short intervals to not overexert

Example 1: 500m row (plug in any cardio activity you wish)

Start 10s slower than your normal pace for 500m, then increase each round by 5 seconds. Repeat for 4-8 sets or until your heart rate spikes rapidly.

Set 1 = 1:45s to complete 500m

Set 2 = 1:40s to complete 500m

Set 3 = 1:35s to complete 500m

Example 2: 15-minute bike interval

Start at a low intensity e.g. 50% of your heart rate maximum. Build from 50% to 85% throughout the intervals. The last 3-5 minutes of the 15-minute block should be hard, but tolerable.

Example 3: weight-based circuit

For our die-hard cardio avoiders that still wish to receive cardio benefits try the following.

1 hour as many rounds as possible (AMRAP):

- 6 x Push-ups

- 6 x Goblet Squats

- 8 x Chin-ups

- 10 cal x Assault bike

- 30 x rope slams

Repeat x 10-15 sets

RESPIRATION LIMITATION

Our last archetype is generally people that may gravitate toward cardio-based activities. These people will benefit from aiming for quality movement, as you will often see they are extended through their thoracic spine with an anterior pelvic tilt (refer to Chapter 3 — Figure 3.2). This archetype is known to compensate through their biomechanics leading to poor breathing mechanics and ultimately a breakdown in their form and performance.

- **Moderate to long intervals** - This will enable them to increase their nervous system output (neural drive) allowing them to gain strength in their required athletic postures.

Example 1: 30-45 minute AMRAP

Cardio activity at 75% max intensity for as long as tolerable.

Example 2: 45-minute AMRAP

500m repeats for as long as comfortable. Resting 90-180 seconds between sets.

DELIVERY / RESPIRATION LIMITATION

Lastly, by now it is evident that everything is rarely black and white when it comes to our anatomy and physiology. If you happen to be a combination of delivery and respiratory limited archetypes you may benefit from the following:

Example 1:

Row at a light to moderate pace, aiming to increase the pace by 5 seconds every 500m until an RPE of 7-8 is achieved.

Rest until 8/10 recovery.

Example 2:

Assault bike at 75% max wattage until breathing or biomechanics are compromised

Rest until complete recovery then starts again.

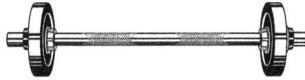

Overview

We have essentially just covered is the first six months of programming for a newbie to training. The flow from programme to programme is essential, and it adds an element of fun (although I do not view this as an essential variable) as well as being engaging and effective to ensure the targeted goals are met with sufficient volume, intensity and specificity to elicit adaptation.

We have created programmes that influence and impact the entire body so the person or you can improve upon the movement capabilities in all fundamental patterns of life. These templates also provided room for variability and individuality as you see fit. We can adapt them with specific exercises, variations and modifications to match what an individual requires, essentially giving them what they lack in order to be capable of doing more with their bodies.

This is a template, a good template that is going to be appropriate for the majority of people reading this book. Now you know the underlying principles, guidelines and recommendations, you should be able to start creating your own programmes.

14

Make Your Cake

"It is health that is the real wealth, and not pieces of gold and silver." -Mahatma Gandhi

We have discussed movement, its variability and the way to elicit adaptation through principles of progressive overload, specificity and time. These are directly related to one pillar of your health, physical activity. There are several other pillars that contribute to your health that I wish to discuss. Just as we should view movement globally, we must adopt a holistic approach when it comes to our overall health. Health is not merely the act of being physically healthy. Instead, it consists of the following pillars:

- Nutrition

- Physical activity

- Sleep

- Stress

To me, these are the four most fundamental aspects that enable us to live a healthy life.

PILLAR 1

NUTRITION

Nutrition is fuel for our bodies. Nutrition, or should I say well-rounded nutrition, can enrich us with energy and regulate our mood. It can help us sustain a variety of physical and mental activities. Conversely, as you can imagine, malnutrition, the act of under nourishing our body, can kill us or seriously harm our physiological systems.

Nutrition, or the act of fuelling oneself, when viewed through the lens of survival, has led to growth, adaptation and travel among species worldwide. Without food, we cease to exist. Now, if we take this a step further and view the physiologic changes that can occur through nutrition, the saying we are what we eat rings true. Throughout our lifetime, a large majority of our cells – those tiny substates that make us, us –die, grow and replenish. This constant turnover encourages healing.

For example, skin cells and red blood cells have a relatively short lifespan, while others like your skeletal cells last up to 10 years. Where do these cells get the energy to keep replenishing and regrowing? Objects cannot be created out of thin air, they come from the transfer of energy. Understand this and you will start to appreciate the power and control a well-rounded diet gives you. We replenish ourselves from what we eat, therefore we become what we eat.

Do you want to choose food sources that have no value, no benefit to the replenishment of your body in one of your key pillars of health and life?

If your answer is no, then keep reading. If you said yes, then still keep reading.

A well-rounded diet involves looking after two key variables, your macronutrients and micronutrients.

The macronutrients, as you may be aware, consist of our protein, carbohydrates and fats. We can manipulate these variables in favour of good health or abuse them and cause ill health. Overindulgence of these macronutrients can lead to conditions such as obesity, diabetes, heart disease and cancers to name a few. A wholesome diet containing appropriate levels of the above can reduce blood pressure, create healthier arteries and adequate body composition and bone density levels throughout your lifespan.

PROTEIN

If you have ever been to a commercial gym, you'll know protein is all the rave. If you have been trained by a personal trainer, they will tell you to eat more protein. Do you know why this is such a renowned and essential macronutrient that is frequently cited among the health and fitness industry?

Protein acts as a catalyst for building not just muscle, but your entire body. Protein can be found within your hair cells, bone and skin, plus it has around 10,000 other functions. We need protein to keep us alive. We use this macronutrient to encourage healthy cell production and even as an energy source (in extreme occasions). Long story short, this macronutrient actually lives up to the hype around it.

In the context of physical activity, our body fluctuates constantly throughout the day, building and breaking down protein. There are two key processes in this alchemy, called muscle protein synthesis (MPS) and muscle protein breakdown (MPB). MPS is the driving force behind our adaption following a training session.

As we train, we stimulate higher MPS than MPB to counteract the toll our training stimulus has on our bodies. This is a good thing because it enables our bodies to grow larger and continue adapting to overcome our environment.

We can manipulate the equilibrium between MPS and MPB in favour through a combination of nutrition and training. Within the context of nutrition, we can eat protein-dense meals regularly throughout our day, with the current recommended range being 1g to 3g per kilogram of body weight.[43,44] This means that if I was 100kg, then I could have between 100g and 300g of protein. Sounds like a lot, right?

This will differ from person to person, with people wishing to build muscle and achieve certain physical feats needing higher quantities of protein, while those looking to maintain their current physical appearance and regulation of their body's mechanisms needing less.

Ultimately, the goal for everyone should be to stay in MPS for as long as we can. Think of the two systems like this:

MPS > MPB = gaining muscle

MPS = MPB: we maintain our lean muscle

MPS< MPB = muscle loss

If you're being trained by me, you'll want to be neutral or in surplus for protein synthesis. We want to reduce MPB but not prevent it. Recent research indicates that reducing total muscle wastage or catabolism by offsetting MPB and stimulating MPS can be beneficial for building muscle. MPB still may have an important role overall in assisting the remodelling of muscle.[45]

How can we tip the scales in favour of MPS?

Training – this increases myofibrillar muscle protein synthesis(muscle-building). Intensities of 70-90% of your one-rep maximum are ideal.

Nutrition – eating well at regular intervals (every three to four hours) can offset MPB and favour anabolism (muscle building).

Basically, if you want to feel good, eat high-quality protein such as eggs or dairy, whey protein supplements and meat (there are alternatives for vegans and vegetarians) while also aiming for regular resistance training at least two or three times per week to stimulate MPS and help develop your muscle.

Now we know adequate ranges and what to do to maintain them. What happens if we fall below this for too long?

Well, this is known as being protein deficient. This issue is not common in Western societies, but it's a problem elsewhere. Worldwide, it is estimated that one billion people or one in seven at the time of writing have some form of protein deficiency.[46] The referenced study indicates that this is particularly prevalent in central Africa and southern Asia. Does this even matter though? Read the effects below, and you tell me!

As well as cancer and anorexia, protein deficiency can cause muscle loss, swelling of the skin (oedema), nail and hair issues, increased risk of infections and greater susceptibility to bone fractures and conditions like osteoporosis to name a few.

This might have you worried, and you may be asking what are proteins exactly? Proteins consist of amino acids, 20 to be precise. Within the context of everyday functioning, we need all 20 amino acids to make protein. Out of the 20, 11 of these amino acids can be regulated through your own body. These are referred to as non-essential amino acids, basically we can make them ourselves. That leaves us with nine essential amino acids that our bodies cannot reproduce, meaning we must source them from somewhere else, e.g., our diet.

All protein is not created equal. Protein sources differ, and it is recommended to reach your required intake through a variety of sources. For example, vegetable-rich proteins such as legumes, nuts and wholegrains are a viable option but not necessarily efficient. Let me explain.

While I do recommend vegetables as a regular source of your protein, vegans and vegetarians should be aware that some of these vegetables will not have a complete amino acid profile. They may have 16 out of the 20, for example, leaving you still requiring four. This is why it is crucial that you develop a plan and map out the profiles of foods if you choose these diets. This will enable you to still get complete profiles to supply your body with sustenance and fuel for your key bodily functions.

For those that aren't veggies, alternative sources such as meat and poultry have complete amino acid profiles and are often cited as complete proteins. Depending on your ethics, religion or taste, you may opt for being vegetarian or vegan. If so, use this as a starting point to understanding what constitutes a healthy diet.

The bottom line is that protein is crucial for building a healthy diet. I will often recommend this macronutrient in regular doses throughout the day. Remember to aim for high-quality protein sources at regular intervals. Research at the time of writing suggests we can only absorb so much, approximately 40g per serving.

So don't consume 100g in one sitting! Break it up and your body will utilise it more efficiently.

FAT

At times I think to myself that the world has a vendetta against fat. Everywhere I turn, media, clients, trainers and the like are trying the newest ways to
obliterate fat. What if I told you fat was vital for keeping you alive?

A certain level of fat is required within our daily diet to promote healthy organ function; organs such as our brain (a pretty important one) thrive from healthy fats. The reason behind this is that the brain is largely constituted of fat! Fat can exist in multiple states, both solid and liquid. Our brain relies on liquid fat to coat our cell membranes, allowing us to have healthy, fluid cells.

The type of fat to include in our diet is another hot topic. There exist multiple types of fats: saturated, unsaturated and trans are the big three, with sub-groups existing within each. What's the difference? you ask.

In a nutshell, the chemical makeup of each type of fat is different. Typically, the more pronounced bad fats will be solid at room temperature, whereas the healthier fats may be liquid at room temperature.

The commonly demonised trans fat sits nicely in the category of being solid at room temperature. This type of fat is included in food to prevent its decay, but unfortunately, the result is that it decays our internal systems, e.g., arteries, instead. This process turns sources of fat that were once healthy into solid forms of fat. The good news is that these are becoming largely banned from food sources. It is now well known that consuming these trans fats has no benefit, but instead they contribute to increases in our 'bad' cholesterol, which is low-density lipoprotein (LDL) cholesterol. LDL cholesterol is actually large, and it collects in our arteries leading to the gradual blockage or stenosis of our interior vein maze. This causes nasty medical conditions including heart disease, stroke and diabetes to name a few. Just in case you weren't aware, cardiovascular diseases are the biggest killers of the human race at the moment. Common sources for our trans-fat foods, I'm afraid to say, are takeaways, baked goods, popcorn and the like.

Healthy fats, commonly referred to as unsaturated fats, can be broken down into further subcategories of polyunsaturated and monounsaturated fats. Common sources for both of these types of healthy fats are nuts, vegetables, seeds and fish to name a few.

Saturated fats were once akin to trans-fat, demonised and believed to cause heart attacks. These days, research points towards saturated fats as not being the worst thing in the world, with no link between saturated fats and increases in heart disease or ill health.[47] There's still no definitive research that determines whether saturated fats, such as those found in cheese, eggs, milk and meat products, should be avoided or included, so at the bare minimum proceed with caution and use in moderation.

Fat is a powerful energy source, particularly for aerobic-based activities. Recommendations about which fat to eat should ideally be made by a qualified professional, such as a nutritionist or dietician. However, if you are trained in nutrition, you can still give valuable dietary advice. It is worth knowing that, per gram, fat contains more calories than proteins and carbohydrates.

EXAMPLE:

100 grams of protein and carbohydrates = 400 calories

100 grams of fat = 900 calories

Fats are satiating. They fill us up, as they are slow to digest, which can be an invaluable tool when aiming for body composition goals. A healthy recommendation of fat is between 25-40% of your total calorie intake. Yes, I know, other diets such as keto opt for a much higher percentage of total calories, so this is case by case.

Look to include good-quality fat from a nice mixture of food sources and you will be on your way to a healthier, happier you! Don't fear it.

CARBOHYDRATES

Is your mouth watering at the sight of the word 'carbs'? Carbohydrates are another misunderstood macronutrient, one that people have claimed to be the sole cause of obesity (not true). In truth, carbohydrates act as one of the most essential energy sources for our bodies, creating readily available energy during aerobic and anaerobic exercise. They are a source of red blood cells and are used for developing the structural components of our cell walls. Carbohydrates come in the form of mouth-watering foods, such as pizza and potatoes, as well as much healthier alternatives, such as fruits, vegetables, legumes and grains.

Within the human body, carbohydrates are broken down into simple molecules called glucose. Glucose is a substrate we can store in our muscles and livers to again supply us with readily available energy and hormone secretion. Hormones such as insulin are useful for transporting glucose out of our bloodstream and into our muscles and liver for energy. Through poor lifestyle choices or autoimmune conditions, such as type 2 and type 1 diabetes mellitus, our body becomes less efficient at utilising or producing insulin, leading to increases in our bloodstream's glucose levels. Still with me?

When these levels of blood glucose are chronically elevated, our body becomes stressed, leading to conditions known as hyperglycaemia. This can damage the vessels that supply the blood to our organs, leading to a potential risk of heart disease, stroke, kidney disease, vision and nerve problems to name a few. Your body basically becomes insulin resistant, diminishing the transportation of glucose out of your body and into the muscles. If you or someone you know is diabetic or has another health condition fitting the criteria, then please seek advice from a qualified dietician or nutritionist regarding the best dietary approach.

This poor management or overconsumption is partly why carbohydrates get such a bad rap. However, they are still a vital energy source for moderate- to high-intensity exercises, basically, those where you don't need too much oxygen. Guidelines suggest that about 30-50% of your total diet should consist of good-quality carbohydrates.

Again, they should be good quality, namely complex carbohydrates (oats and pasta) mostly, with some simple carbohydrates. Avoid sugar (simple carbs), difficult I know as it is in a copious number of foods these days. It gives you no real value other than a quick spike in your glucose levels.

Now, I know fruit has sugar so you're probably wondering if that is bad. The answer is no.

Fruits with decent fibre content (3-5g per serving) are ideal. This is because fibre slows down the rate of absorption of sugar; in other words, it doesn't stimulate a panic response from your pancreas to secrete insulin to calm the glucose. Instead, this is a slow and steady release, allowing for better absorption and a reduced toll on your metabolism. I prefer blending over juicing for this reason. Juicing gets rid of the skin, seeds and pulp, in other words the fibre-containing properties, so it gives you a spike in glucose. You've been warned!

If you are still unsure about what dietary advice to offer someone, you have a few options. Either become qualified by educating yourself through reputable courses or ask an expert e.g., dieticians and nutritionists. A poor diet is akin to overtraining:

it can wreak havoc on your body and mess up multiple vital processes that allow you to function.

So, if you are relatively healthy and want to start altering your intake of macronutrients, you will need to form some habits and create the environment to achieve success. To do this, we need a look at a few variables.

- Your current weight – this is our starting point.

- Your target weight – we can set percentages to determine how aggressive your approach will be.

- Your activity level – this must be accounted for to ensure you are eating enough calories.

Now I will provide a few macro-based and habit-based examples so you can understand how the approaches may differ and why they may be suitable for different demographics.

MACRO-BASED EXAMPLES

When determining your macronutrient recommendations using the above information, we want to determine your basal metabolic rate (BMR). This is a fancy way of saying what you can currently eat every single day based on the above variables and not gain or lose weight. BMR is simply the calories we require to keep our bodies alive, our organs functioning. People much smarter than me have figured out a multitude of ways to track this through complex formulas. To date, two of the most accurate ways I'm aware of are the Mifflin-St Jeor and Harris Benedict equations. The following is based on Mifflin-St Jeor.[48]

$$BMR \text{ (kcal/day)} = 10 * weight \text{ (kg)} + 6.25 * height \text{ (cm)} - 5 * age \text{ (yr)} + 5 \text{ (kcal/day)}$$

EXAMPLE: A 25-YEAR-OLD MALE WEIGHING 80KG, 180CM TALL

$(10 * 80) + (6.25 * 180) - (5 * 25) + 5 = 1{,}805$ calories per day.

The above gives you a resting energy expenditure level i.e., how much you would burn without movement. I'm assuming you are going to move because you're reading this book so, please factor in the activity factor, i.e., how much you move across the week approximately.

· 1.2 = Sedentary (desk job, little formal exercise)

· 1.3-1.4 = Lightly Active (light daily activity AND light exercise one to three days a week)

· 1.5-1.6 = Moderately Active (moderate daily activity and moderate exercise three to five days a week)

· 1.7-1.8 = Very Active (physically demanding lifestyle and hard exercise six to seven days a week)

· 1.9-2.2 = Extremely Active (Athlete in endurance training or doing a very hard physical job)

If we take our above BMR of 1,805 and times it by 1.2 for a sedentary office worker, we get 2,166 kcal/day.

If we instead use someone who is moderately active and times it by 1.6, we get a value of 2,888 kcal/day.

As you can see, it is essential to account for activity to get a more accurate representation of what a person can eat while still losing weight. Be honest with yourself; if in doubt about your activity level, go with the lower options initially.

Now, once we have determined the BMR of the individual I recommend doing the following:

1. Measure body weight longitudinally – this means weighing yourself several times a week and calculating the average. This is not the most accurate measure, but it is still meaningful data when taken repeatedly. For example, measure yourself on Monday, Wednesday, Friday, and Saturday instead of just once per week.

2. Monitor fluctuations for at least two weeks before altering your approach. Even after two weeks, ensure you are hitting your metrics for training intensity, consistency, sleeping and other factors of nutrition before increasing or decreasing your calorie intake for the day.

3. Use percentages, not generic numbers. Simply put, it is more accurate to use 10% of your total daily energy expenditure (TDEE) instead of simply reducing intake by 500 calories.

4. Understand your end goal and timeframe so you know when to stop, how aggressive to be with your approach and what exactly you are aiming for.

Using our above example of the 25-year-old, let's look at some possible weight-loss and muscle-growth scenarios.

Example 1: Weight Loss

Sedentary person: 2166 kcal/day – 10% TDE = 1,949 kcal/day

Active person: 2,888 kcal/day – 10% TDE = 2,599 kcal/day

Example 2: Hypertrophy

Sedentary person: 2,166 kcal/day + 15% TDE = 2,490 kcal/day

Active person: 2,888 kcal/day + 15% TDE = 3,321 kcal/day

The differences between these are vast. If I was to simply use a generic number of 500 calories per day instead, for example, you may be in an unfavourable position to lose weight, one where the process is too fast and you begin to lose other valuable areas such as lean muscle mass.

Another issue that may arise is psychological fatigue. Preventing someone from eating their normal diet affects more than just their physical body. The psychological stress should be understood and accounted for throughout any dieting. By using a diet percentage ranging between 10% and 30% (30 only for short periods) we can carefully manipulate the calories in a way that is specific and tailored to the needs of the individual person and relative data.

Now we have determined the daily calories required for the above examples, we need to break this down into their macronutrients (protein, carbs and fats).

Protein recommendations

Protein, as previously mentioned, ranges from a recommended dose of 1g/kg to 3g/kg per day. For a 100kg person, this means a whopping variance of 100g to 300g. I will generally opt for a percentage of their daily intake and allocate this to each of their macros. For protein, again depending on the person and their goals, I will allocate between 25% to 40% of their total calories.

To work this out, I set ranges. Let's take a client with a range between 25% and 30% of their total daily intake.

Sedentary hypertrophy client's total daily intake = 2,490 calories

Protein = 25% of 2,490 = 622.5 calories

622.5/4 (calories in a gram of protein) = 156g of protein/day

Protein = 30% of 2,490 = 747

747/4 = 187g of protein/day

This gives us a range of 156-187g. For the vast majority, this range will be sufficient; for those with specific goals, we might have a smaller range of 25%-27.5%, for example.

FAT RECOMMENDATIONS

Next, I will determine their fat needs for each day. Again, our ranges will typically be between 25-35% of their daily intake. The below example is for a range of 25-30%, again for our sedentary person.

25% of 2,490 = 622.5

622.5/9 (calories per gram) = 69g of fat

30% of 2,490 = 747

747/9 = 83g of fat

Our range for fat is 69-83g per day.

Carbohydrate recommendations

Lastly, carbs. Since we have already allocated approximately 50-60% of our total daily intake, we will work out our carbohydrates based on 40-50% (high carbs).

40% of 2,490 = 996 calories

996/4 (calories per gram) = 249g of carbohydrates

50% of 2,490 = 1,245 calories

1,245/4 = 311g of carbohydrates

Our range for carbs is 249-311g per day.

This makes up our total calories of 2,490 for the person.

Protein = 156-187g/day (624-748 calories)

Fat = 69-83g/day (621-747 calories)

Carbs = 249-311g/day (996-1,244 calories)

Now, if we were to go the high end for each of their macros, we would place people at a disadvantage by increasing their total calories by roughly 250 per day. This is obviously not ideal. It's a case of give and take. If we have higher variability for some macro targets, we must take it from the other macro nutrients.

Overall, using a range is much more sustainable and less stressful psychologically compared to hitting a fixed number every day.

HABIT-BASED APPROACH

This is a method I find particularly useful for people that do not wish to track, are new to tracking, simply don't understand tracking well enough or are chronic dieters.

Habit-based approaches allow us to select areas of their diet and give them habits, specific areas to focus on to improve their outcomes in this part of their diet. This may come in the form of increasing their protein around breakfast, eating 'x' number of servings of vegetables, or avoiding unhealthy foods at certain times. This develops understanding of what constitutes a well-rounded diet without becoming too focused on numbers. This can be just as successful for people improving their health. Typically, this is best accompanied by adherence tracking sheets. These sheets will enable the client, and the trainer, to view objectively how well they can stick to the plan.

This can still be used in conjunction with our macro-based approach, in fact it will improve results. Forming habits is a way to make lasting behavioural changes. Equipping people with the tools to understand what they are eating, why they are eating it and what is too much or too little means they can become independent and change their behaviours themselves.

In contrast, diets involving preprepared meals, while convenient, often do not create lasting change, or should I say are not as effective. This is because there's no education involved, therefore once someone stops, they go back to the habits that led them to need a diet in the first place. A vicious cycle, you might call it; one built on dependence rather than growth and independence. Choose independence and educate yourself about healthy diets.

In my experience, the more specific we get with our goals, the more specific our training and nutrition must become. For most people who want to have more energy, feel better about themselves and improve their body composition, habit-based approaches are effective. For those who have other goals of competing in body-building competitions, athletic events or those with health conditions, we must fine-tune our macro-advice and give them specific breakdowns of what they require.

With any diet, we must think in terms of moderation and have a clear date for when we will cease. As a rule of thumb, keep your dieting periods under 12 weeks otherwise the psychological stress and fatigue will take too much of a toll.

PILLAR 2

PHYSICAL ACTIVITY

The guidelines for physical activity should be well understood by now. They are in place to maintain the quality of your health. If we wish to reap the benefits of exercise, we must meet these guidelines throughout all stages of our lives.

Physical activity will help you become healthy. This is a fundamental pillar as it keeps us youthful. Given the right dosage of physical activity medicine, we can prevent and manage a large number of age-related declines – osteoporosis, dementia and arthritis to name a few.

A combined approach Combining resistance training with aerobic exercise is often found to be the most successful way to implement an exercise regime.[49]

The basis of this book is physical activity, so by now we should be well-versed in how and why we must exercise throughout all stages of our life.

As a quick refresher, aim to meet the following guidelines:

Low to moderate exercise of 150-300 minutes per week. The frequency is important here. Aim to move in some capacity daily! Walk, run, swim – you get the drift.

OR

Vigorous activity of 75-120 minutes per week. This can be less frequent due to the taxing demands. Aim to move through HITT workouts, sprinting and mowing the lawn.

For resistance training, we want to aim for at least two or three sessions for the whole body per week on top of the previous cardiovascular. The more trained you are, the more you may need to continue adapting.

PILLAR 3

SLEEP

Asking why sleep may be a pillar of health is akin to asking why we need oxygen to survive. We would die faster from sleep deprivation than we would from food deprivation. Read that again.

Without sleep, our pain tolerance is reduced, leading to an almost hyper sensitive state where pain and our perceived effort is altered.

There's a reason we spend a third of our lives asleep, or at least we should. And it's not just vital for humans. Sleep is needed by every species throughout the world.

It's recommended we sleep for seven to nine hours on average, however this does change based on different age groups. Studies have highlighted some alarming facts around lack of sleep, with some research reporting the reaction times of a person that has been awake for 24 hours to be equivalent of someone legally drunk.[50,51]

Poor sleep also impairs recovery following a training session, which has obvious implications for injury risk and performance outcomes.[52]

It even affects hormones such as leptin and ghrelin, which are important for regulating how much we eat, and how we feel after eating.[53]

The bottom line is sleep is important. Lack of sleep has been linked with a multitude of both physical and mental health conditions. Its importance is sometimes lost in our modern, fast-paced world. We are the only species that sacrifice our sleep. Sleep should be non-negotiable, something we put above all else for our survival, and yet we don't.

By now, you have probably thought of your own reasons for giving up sleep: seeing friends, work, watching Netflix, cramming for exams to name a few.

We can greatly improve our quality of life by adopting a few simple sleeping habits. When looking to help someone in this regard, I will often try to understand their sleep ritual. This refers to the processes, behaviours and activities they undergo prior to getting into bed. This may include how they eat before bed, how they entertain themselves, whether they exercise close to their bedtime. I will often present this to them in the form of a tracking sheet, similar to the one I'd use to measure their daily diet; a sleep recall, if you will. I use this questionnaire to understand their regular and irregular activities, things that can help or hinder their slumber.

One of the main problems is technology use – think smartphones, televisions, tablets and computers. Do you use any of these before you sleep?

When using this form of technology, blue light is emitted. This is high-frequency light and energy source which blocks hormones like melatonin from being released to our brain to initiate the process of us falling asleep. In an ideal situation, the melatonin hormone is released a few hours prior to sleeping, allowing us to cool our core temperature down and drift into the abyss of sleep once we close our eyes and rest our head. When the hormone is blocked or reduced via blue light, it's more difficult to sleep.

If you are someone who scrolls through Facebook or watches TV until you fall asleep, I recommend using the built-in blue-light filters that exist on all your smart devices a few hours before bedtime. These block out the blue light and give you a yellow tinge on your screens. Personally, I use this filter from 5 pm; I just set it on repeat and forget, job done. This way you can still perform the same activities but with less inhibition of melatonin.

How dark is your bedroom? This, along with temperature, can be make or break for getting a healthy amount of sleep. If lamps or streetlights flood your bedroom with light, or it's too hot, it can be quite difficult to fall asleep. Make sure you block all external light sources and open a window or use a fan or aircon to bring the temperature down throughout the room/house. If you are really dedicated, you can look to devices like the 'ChiliPAD' that basically cools your bed to an ideal temperature through water tubes. This allows you to monitor the temperature of your bed with high accuracy. An ideal temperature for our bodies to drift into sleep is 18-20 degrees Celsius.[54,55]

Some people may have difficulty 'switching off', an ever-increasing issue in today's hectic society. We are bombarded with constant notifications, light, noise and thoughts. The act of being mindful is forgotten for some at night. This leads to overthinking and replaying the past day's events, or planning what is to come in the upcoming days.

Have you ever tried brushing your teeth with your non-dominant hand? Overthinking at night is just as stimulating for the brain as this unusual pattern, making it extremely difficult to fall asleep. Now, it is obviously easier said than done to just switch off our minds. Depending on the person I am working with, I may encourage them to try journaling — looking at key upcoming events and prioritising them in order of crucial, important, non-important and miscellaneous. This can enable and encourage sleep by simply getting thoughts out of their head and onto paper. Other strategies include meditation to practise letting thoughts come and go, reading or watching light movies, even having a ban on technology for those who are glued to their phones. Hopefully, these ideas will spark some other ideas about how you can get the rest you deserve.

PILLAR 4

STRESS

If there is one thing I know for certain, it is that stress is an unavoidable, inevitable part of your life. Every day, each living being on this planet will encounter stress. It may come in the form of looking for food, finding somewhere to sleep, studying for a test, paying bills, parking, meeting deadlines, training or watching the latest episode of your favourite TV show. All of these elicit a form of stress, good or bad.

Why is stress so shunned in society?

Countless books and articles have been written (the irony in writing this) on stress and how to avoid it.

Let's first understand what stress is, what it does to us and why everyone is afraid of it.

Stress can occur in a multitude of ways, including physical, psychological, behavioural and environmental. When we sense stress, our body taps into the sympathetic nervous system. As we have discussed, has a number of physiological effects, increasing our blood pressure and respiratory rate and priming our nervous and musculature systems to give us the best chance to overcome whatever we face.

Now, in small doses this is healthy; it's when we move into the realm of chronic stress that we start to tread a dangerous path. Stress, or should I say chronic stress, will increase our susceptibility to mood disorders, cardiovascular events like heart attacks and strokes and conditions such as post-traumatic stress disorder (PTSD).

On a day-to-day basis, we will not only encounter stress within ourselves but cue to the people we encounter. These people, like you, will have multifactorial stressors – kids, work, bills, sleep deprivation and so on. Understanding this can teach you a valuable lesson in empathy and relating to those around you. Stress impacts every facet of our being. Being stressed can impair your thoughts, emotional intelligence and emotional regulation. As well as your performance in work or recreational activities. I like to visualise this concept as a plate of food. If I had a normal-sized plate, and I just keep piling on more and more food, eventually it will spill over. Things fall off at random. In reality, this might mean an argument with your significant other, it may cause you to neglect your health, miss your kid's sports day, forget about feeding your dog and so on. Stress must be balanced.

We know that training is another stress. Knowing when and when not to apply stress is a skill and a balancing act. Someone who is used to juggling hundreds of activities may be able to chuck training into the mix, whereas another person may struggle with just 10 activities. This is where periodising your training comes in handy. If you realise that there will be times when your plate is full, you can tailor your needs around this. Remember, it's a bit of give and take. If you focus more on one area of your life, focus less on another so that your stress levels stay balanced.

So, what should we do with stress?

Rather than cower or try to avoid stress (which can actually cause more stress), we should embrace it, accept it, understand it and learn how to use it to our advantage.

Below is my step-by-step guide to understanding and utilising stress.

1.Recognise your stressed

Sounds simple, but for most people stress goes unnoticed, that is until it becomes evident throughout their body. People may have increased muscle tone/tightness, trouble falling asleep, concentration issues, feel irritable. Biting your nails or shaking your leg excessively, even clenching your jaw, are common symptoms. The ways stress can present can be subtle, so pay attention!

2. Understand your triggers

Now we are aware that we have stress, it is time to understand what steps, stressors or events led us to this stressful state. Are there particular things, like a messy house or your boss pilin g on the work tasks, that led you to feel this way? Jot down a list of potential pet hates that make your blood boil.

3. Figure out what you can change

So, now you have some idea about what triggers are stressing you out. The next step is making a change, look at the low-hanging fruits and triggers that are changeable right now.

- With nutrition, this can involve focusing on one key task that is either easy enough to accomplish or that will impact other areas.

- The easy tasks give you momentum, and the one that impacts other areas will help you manage your stress more effectively.

- An example could be to realise you are failing to get more than five hours' sleep on your weekdays. Make changing this a priority and you may see an improvement in your mood and your ability to handle the workload and deal with others.

4. Make a plan

- Unfortunately, we can't change all our stressors but that doesn't mean we can't get ready for them. By understanding our previous triggers, we will know more accurately when to expect certain types of stress e.g., work, bills and interactions with certain people.

- This allows us to pre-empt our stress by visualising what it would be like. By theoretically 'living' through the stress in this way, we can help take the edge off when we actually experience it.

5. Keep things simple

Stress takes away simplicity; we forget to smell the roses and instead focus on the storm in front of us. This is a cue to slow down, and have something handy that is calming or thought-provoking to bring you back to the present moment. For me, when I'm overly stressed, I will listen to some of my favourite music. Other options may involve meditating, grounding, art, and watching movies. Basically, tap into that not-so-serious right side of your brain.

6. Move your body

- Remember, stress is not created equal. Time to utilise some of that stress through controlled doses of movement. This type of stress is healthy; it may mitigate your unhealthy stress by clearing your head, increasing blood flow to your muscles and joints, releasing endorphins (natural mood-enhancing chemicals) and boosting your overall energy levels.

- Low-energy activities like walking can be an easy way to reduce your overall stress while not placing you under more. It's a lot easier to go for a walk than perform hill sprints when you're stressed – create an environment for success!

Feel better yet?

Overview

Pillars of Health

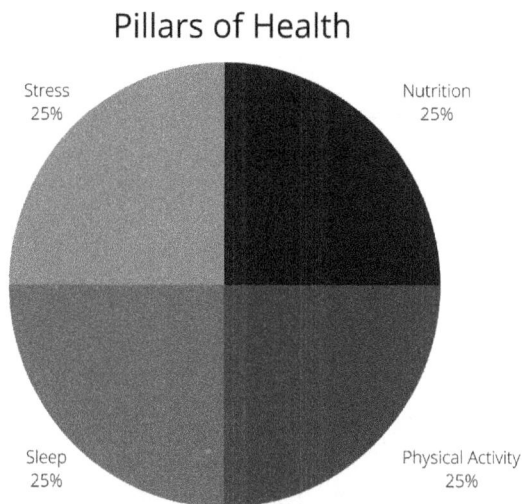

Figure 14.1

This pie chart, equally divided into four segments, shows that each of these pillars is essential; each should be understood, respected and maintained to ensure we have a quality lifestyle that allows us to complete any task we set out to. By neglecting part of our pie chart, we neglect our health.

If you intend to either help yourself or others, you must give each pillar the attention it deserves. Each one is as essential as the other; placing too much emphasis on one will lead to damage over time. Without adequate nutrition, we won't have the energy for a decent training session. Without a decent training session, we won't elicit the adaptations and growth we are after. Without sleep, we will not recover and therefore again fail to adapt to our stimulus, leading to stress. Without mitigating our stress, we will inevitably burn out, lack consistency of effort in our chosen areas of life and our risk of disease will increase. It is a vicious cycle, yet a very manageable one.

Another approach I use to keep a balance between the pillars is to allocate a simple point system to this process. Let's say you have 10 points for your week. Once you score all 10 points that's it, no more. Each category of nutrition, physical activity, sleep and stress must be allocated at least one point.

We can only allocate so many points to each category. If we give four to nutrition, four to training and one each to sleep and stress, we will be at an imbalance. At times this will change throughout your life, but ideally aim to allocate two or three points to each category. Use this as a guide to how well you control your pillars of health!

15

Don't Wait Till Monday

"The path to success is to take massive, determined actions." - Tony Robbins

L et this final chapter serve as an overview, an amalgamation of all the concepts we have discussed throughout the book. Below I've summarised the previous chapters into a short digestible read. This can be used for reflection, as a way to stimulate your thoughts and something to come back to when you need to consolidate.

Breathing is one of the most powerful ways to change yourself, period. Breathing is the raw pattern regulating our bodily systems, influencing our movement, nervous system and mindset. To create lasting change in any endeavour related to our body's physiology, we must incorporate breathing in a conscious, controlled manner.

Locomotion is complex: we are not machines, rather we are a collection of multifaceted patterns working in synergy to propel us forward and keep us alive. Remember to adopt a holistic approach to movement incorporating all three planes of motion. This is essential if you are to capture the entirety of your movement capabilities.

Preparation in the form of warming up and cooling down will enable us to heighten our physiology when we need it most, before bringing it back down to allow sufficient recovery. To assess what we need within our programmes we must carry out repeatable, valid testing measures to get an idea of how our body works as a whole. From here we can engage with the essential preparatory exercises aimed at providing sensory stimulation to encourage postural changes and improved movement capacity. This should focus on the whole self – thinking about the biological, psychological and social aspects and the relevance of each to you at different times. This will allow you to alter the stimulus you require, your beliefs when necessary and the social aspects you may need to engage with less or more.

To move requires stability and mobility. Without stability, we lack mobility and vice versa. Each joint should have the capacity to be stable and mobile in differing contexts. The body is rarely affected globally without leading to compensation in another region. Our body is incredibly adaptive; we can adopt alternative patterns in order to compensate for a lack of stability and mobility in particular areas. Short-term this can be great, long term not so much.

To improve our body, we must follow certain principles. These principles exist all around us, governing us and maintaining order. Within the context of training, the FITT principles and progressive overload, reversibility, adaptation, recovery and exercise selection are inseparable from getting results.

Understanding the patterns that developed throughout evolution and fine-tuned during the first stages of our life gives us insight into our movement today! This is commonly seen at the gym in movements of pushing, pulling, carrying, squatting and hinging, helping make our lives seamless in all planes of motion.

Once we understand the principles and patterns, we can venture into the creative realm of programming methodologies. These allow us to manipulate variables of repetitions, volume, intensity, tempo and rest, as well as give us scope in how to achieve specific adaptations within our energy systems. Methodologies are in the eye of the beholder: knowing where we are going with our goals and what principles to obey can create limitless approaches to achieving the outcomes.

This process of evolving into our best state, reaching our goal or accomplishing a feat, will be most successful through a methodical, periodised approach. Our periodisation factors in our lifestyle through manipulation of macro, meso and micro training cycles. A good periodisation block will involve peaking and tapering to enable you to reach your best at the right time.

To change movement, the mind has to be conscious. By understanding placebos, noceboes, the power of belief and how to live a life of growth rather than being in a fixed state, we can alter ourselves from within. Wiring and unwiring are skills that we can learn to become versatile, robust, change-oriented creatures. A crucial element of altering your mindset is to self-reflect on past, present and future beliefs regularly. This will enable you to use what works, and remove what no longer serves you.

Now we have the understanding of what it takes to develop, create change, manage behaviours and empathise with people. There are various ways we can communicate. We must engage with people at their level, and meet them with their style of learning so they can understand our language. This is the secret to healthy communication. We have two eyes and ears and only one mouth. This tells us that we should listen, watch and communicate with our body more than we speak. Having the resources to communicate our message will enable meaningful relationships with those around us!

The key to a good programme lies in the variables we include. Goal setting, individualisation, balance, appropriateness and getting the dosage right is essential.

Goal setting should be clear, realistic and scheduled, and there needs to be a rationale behind why we are trying to achieve this. The barriers along the way can be overcome by understanding where we currently sit within the transtheoretical model of behavioural change and what is required to transition through the stages to reach our goal.

When we begin to periodise our programme to achieve our set goals, start with what you need. Introducing yourself towards large bilateral and unilateral programmes as you progress through your training abilities. The first few months of your training life should revolve around learning how to use the body to its capacity rather than just stacking on weight. That comes later as we get more advanced, when we can look towards overloading and utilising more difficult principles and methods.

The intention of all our programmes and advice should be to create our healthiest, wholesome selves. To accomplish this, we have to include the pillars of health, our training, sleep, nutrition and stress. These concepts can be the difference between making or breaking not only our training programmes but our health and wellbeing overall. Our theoretical toolbox should include a range of methods and metrics to understand, evaluate and measure the data that is constantly being given to us on a daily basis – ranging from aches and pains to levels of energy. Once you are aware of your baseline within the four pillars you can take actionable steps to create change.

Ok, take a breath. That was a lot! The final question remains. Now we have this knowledge, what exactly do we do with it?

Don't wait till Monday!

Many of us will fall into the classic trap of putting things off: "Meh, I'll get to that on Monday." Monday then becomes Tuesday, Tuesday becomes the weekend. Before you know it, you've done nothing and it's 32 years later.

Some of you will fall into a personality archetype that relies on procrastination, others may simply be unsure of how to implement change. A simple strategy for helping me get started on any project is to zoom out.

Take a moment and type 'Star Size Comparison' into Google. For me, this serves as a reminder of the big-picture concept. This helps me to overcome any procrastination.

Zooming out allows you to look at that big mountain ahead in your journey towards a healthier you. Next, you start to zoom back in so you can choose a path to tackle this mountain. If you're still stuck, go back to the beginning of the book and start with your goal! This mountain won't climb itself, so it's best you do something immediately after you put this book down!

A simple task could be one of the following:

- Jotting down some large macro goals on your phone or in your journal.

- Going for a walk to think through your plan of attack for starting.

- Putting reminders in your phone.

- Searching related topics that this book may have sparked your interest in on the internet or research portals such as Google Scholar.

- Piecing together a gym programme that can be started today! This doesn't have to be perfect (a programme rarely is) but it could be built on the foundations laid in this book.

- Get an accountability buddy – a family member or friend that will check in on you and your progress.

Like our new year's resolution setters, don't fall into the trap of waiting for Monday. Time is of the essence. By making it this far, you have already proved to yourself that you are committed to becoming the best version of yourself, to climbing your mountain of a goal and achieving success in your life.

I hope you found enjoyment and knowledge from the concepts within this book. These are ones I have discovered through my own research, and I will endeavour to continually update my knowledge and quench my insatiable thirst for learning more. I implore you to do the same: find your passion and follow it unequivocally. Thank you for the time you spent reading this work, may it be of use to you and those around you!

END

References

This section contains any and all references and citations I have used for each chapter as appropriate. I have said multiple times throughout the book that concepts evolve. Some evidence will bolster what I said through and some may refute it. I'm not perfect. Remember, this book should serve as a guide not gospel.

If new information comes to pass or I have just straight up made mistakes throughout the book, tap into my growth mindset and shoot me an email! You can reach me at moverightep@gmail.com. I will amend the issue for future prints

Chapter 1: Compression & Expansion

1. Russo, M. A., Santarelli, D. M., & O'Rourke, D. (2017). The physiological effects of slow breathing in the healthy human. Breathe, 13(4), 298–309. https://doi.org/10.1183/20734735. 009817

2. Zaccaro, A., Piarulli, A., Laurino, M., Garbella, E., Menicucci, D., Neri, B., & Gemignani, A. (2018). How Breath-Control Can Change Your Life: A Systematic Review on Psycho-Physiolog-

ical Correlates of Slow Breathing. Frontiers in Human Neuro-
science, 12(353). https://doi.org/10.3389/fnhum.2018.00353

Chapter 2: Repeat After Me – You Aren't a Terminator

3. Umberger, B. R. (2010). Stance and swing phase costs in
human walking. Journal of the Royal Society Interface, 7(50),
1329–1340. https://doi.org/10.1098/rsif.2010.0084

4. Boyer, K. A., & Hafer, J. F. (2019). Gait mechanics contribute
to exercise induced pain flares in knee osteoarthritis. BMC Musculoskeletal Disorders, 20(1). https://doi.org/10.1186/s12891
-019-2493-4

5. Boss, G. R., & Seegmiller, J. E. (1981). Age-Related
Physiological Changes and Their Clinical Significance. Western
Journal of Medicine, 135(6), 434–440. Retrieved from
https://www.ncbi.nlm.nih.gov/pmc/articles/PMC1273316/#:
~:text=Physiological%20changes%20occur%20with%20aging

6. Kennedy, S. (2017). The Biomechanics of Running:
Understanding the many variables can help prevent or treat
injuries. *Podiatry Management*, [online] 36(7), pp.125–129.
Available at:
https://web.p.ebscohost.com/ehost/detail/detail?vid=7&sid=9
4cb0270-a6c9-4691-b5b1-37d97fbe4680%40redis&bdata=Jn
NpdGU9ZWhvc3QtbGl2ZQ%3d%3d#AN=124995357&db=
ccm.

7. Landreneau, L. L., Watts, K., Heitzman, J. E., & Childers, W.
L. (2014). Lower Limb Muscle Activity During Forefoot and
Rearfoot Strike Running Techniques. International Journal of
Sports Physical Therapy, 9(7), 888–897. Retrieved from
https://web.p.ebscohost.com/ehost/detail/detail?vid=10&sid=

94cb0270-a6c9-4691-b5b1-37d97fbe4680%40redis&bdata=Jn
NpdGU9ZWhvc3QtbGl2ZQ%3d%3d#AN=101816209&db=
s3h

8. Souza, R. B. (2016). An Evidence-Based Videotaped Running
Biomechanics Analysis. Physical Medicine and Rehabilitation
Clinics of North America, 27(1), 217–236. https://doi.org/10
.1016/j.pmr.2015.08.006

9. Cheung, R. T. H., An, W. W., Au, I. P. H., Zhang, J. H., Chan,
Z. Y. S., & MacPhail, A. J. (2018). Control of impact loading
during distracted running before and after gait retraining in
runners. Journal of Sports Sciences, 36(13), 1497–1501.
Retrieved from
https://web.p.ebscohost.com/ehost/pdfviewer/pdfviewer?vid=
3&sid=2531b094-2940-461e-8c9b-bbe8e7f5585a%40redis

10. Wang, B., Yang, Y., Zhang, X., Wang, J., Deng, L., & Fu, W.
(2020). Twelve-Week Gait Retraining Reduced Patellofemoral
Joint Stress during Running in Male Recreational Runners.
BioMed Research International, 2020, 1–9. https://doi.org/1
0.1155/2020/9723563

11. Kennedy, S. (2017). The Biomechanics of Running:
Understanding the many variables can help prevent or treat
injuries. Podiatry Management, [online] 36(7), pp.125–129.
Available at:
https://web.p.ebscohost.com/ehost/detail/detail?vid=7&sid=9
4cb0270-a6c9-4691-b5b1-37d97fbe4680%40redis&bdata=Jn
NpdGU9ZWhvc3QtbGl2ZQ%3d%3d#AN=124995357&db=
ccm.

12. Sung Joong Kim, & JaeHo Yu. (2015). Changes of Gait
Parameters and Lower Limb Dynamics in Recreational
Runners with Achilles Tendinopathy. Journal of Sports Science
& Medicine, 14(2), 284–289. Retrieved from
https://web.p.ebscohost.com/ehost/detail/detail?vid=21&sid=

94cb0270-a6c9-4691-b5b1-37d97fbe4680%40redis&bdata=Jn
NpdGU9ZWhvc3QtbGl2ZQ%3d%3d#AN=102832261&db=
rss

Chapter 3: Preparation Is Success

13. Chorley, A. (2016). The effects of prior post-activation potentiation on 4 km cycling time trial performance. *Sport & Exercise Scientist*, (48), 24–24. Retrieved from https://web.p.ebscohost.com/ehost/detail/detail?vid=2&sid=66545e58-92e0-4d28-99da-b31a5cb20851%40redis&bdata=JnNpdGU9ZWhvc3QtbGl2ZQ%3d%3d#AN=116301136&db=s3h

14. Shrier, I. (2000). Stretching before exercise: an evidence-based approach. British Journal of Sports Medicine, 34(5), 324–325. https://doi.org/10.1136/bjsm.34.5.324

15. Chiba, I., Samukawa, M., Takizawa, K., Nishikawa, Y., Ishida, T., Kasahara, S., ... Tohyama, H. (2022). Warm-Up Intensity and Time-Course Effects on Jump Height under Cold Conditions. International Journal of Environmental Research and Public Health, 19(9), 5781. https://doi.org/10.3390/ijerph19095781

16. Eken, Ö. (2022). The Acute Effect of Different Specific Warm-up Phases on 1- Repetition Maximum Bench Press Results. Pakistan Journal of Medical and Health Sciences, 16(1), 430–433. https://doi.org/10.53350/pjmhs22161430

17. Suh, S.-H., Paik, I.-Y., & Jacobs, K. (2007). Regulation of blood glucose homeostasis during prolonged exercise. Molecules and Cells, 23(3), 272–279. Retrieved from https://web.p.ebscohost.com/ehost/detail/detail?vid=12&sid=66545e58-92e0-4d28-99da-b31a5cb20851%40redis&bdata=JnNpdGU9ZWhvc3QtbGl2ZQ%3d%3d#AN=17646701&db=mdc

18. Martin, B. J., Robinson, S., Wiegman, D. L., & Aulick, L. H. (1975). Effect of warm-up on metabolic responses to strenuous exercise. Medicine and Science in Sports, 7(2), 146–149. Retrieved from https://europepmc.org/article/med/1152628

19. Padua, E., D'Amico, A. G., Alashram, A., Campoli, F., Romagnoli, C., Lombardo, M., ... Annino, G. (2019). Effectiveness of Warm-Up Routine on the Ankle Injuries Prevention in Young Female Basketball Players: A Randomized Controlled Trial. Medicina, 55(10), 690. https://doi.org/10.3390/medicina55100690

20. Parks, J. C., Marshall, E. M., Humm, S. M., Erb, E. K., & Kingsley, J. D. (2022). Effects of a Cool-Down after Supramaximal Interval Exercise on Autonomic Modulation. International Journal of Environmental Research and Public Health, 19(9), 5407. https://doi.org/10.3390/ijerph19095407

21. Clausen, B. (2016). Neuromuscular exercise as treatment for knee osteoarthritis in middle aged patients. *Undefined*. Retrieved from https://www.semanticscholar.org/paper/Neuromuscular-exercise-as-treatment-for-knee-inClausen/f6b54c5d77a177ed014c07fea4fe9a010ed070a6?p2df

Chapter 4: Stability Vs. Mobility (Ding, Ding)

22. Hodges, P. W., Gurfinkel, V. S., Brumagne, S., Smith, T. C., & Cordo, P. C. (2002). Coexistence of stability and mobility in postural control: evidence from postural compensation for respiration. Experimental Brain Research, 144(3), 293–302. https://doi.org/10.1007/s00221-002-1040-x

23. Chandola, T., Brunner, E., & Marmot, M. (2006). Chronic stress at work and the metabolic syndrome: prospective study. BMJ, 332(7540), 521–525. https://doi.org/10.1136/bmj.38693.435301.80

24. Dias-Ferreira, E., Sousa, J. C., Melo, I., Morgado, P., Mesquita, A. R., Cerqueira, J., ... Sousa, N. (2009). Chronic Stress Causes Frontostriatal Reorganization and Affects Decision-Making. Science, 325(5940), 621–625. https://doi.org/10.1126/science.1171203

25. Marin, M.-F., Lord, C., Andrews, J., Juster, R.-P., Sindi, S., Arsenault-Lapierre, G., Lupien, S. J. (2011). Chronic stress, cognitive functioning and mental health. Neurobiology of Learning and Memory, 96(4), 583–595. https://doi.org/10.1016/j.nlm.2011.02.016

Chapter 5: Learn Thy Principles

26. American College of Sports Medicine, Swain, D., & Brawner, C. (2014). ACSM's Resource Manual for Guidelines for Exercise Testing and Prescription. Human Movement Sciences Faculty Books. Retrieved from https://digitalcommons.odu.edu/hms_books/3/

Chapter 6: Motion Is Lotion

27. Kobesova, A., & Kolar, P. (2014). Developmental kinesiology: three levels of motor control in the assessment and treatment of the motor system. Journal of Bodywork and Movement Therapies, 18(1), 23–33. https://doi.org/10.1016/j.jbmt.2013.04.002

Chapter 7: Creating a Mona Lisa

28. Guimarães-Ferreira, L. (2014). Role of the phosphocreatine system on energetic homeostasis in skeletal and cardiac muscles. Einstein (São Paulo), 12(1), 126–131. https://doi.org/10.1590/s1679-45082014rb2741

29. Sahlin, K., Harris, R. C., & Hultman, E. (1979). Resynthesis

of creatine phosphate in human muscle after exercise in relation to intramuscular pH and availability of oxygen. Scandinavian Journal of Clinical and Laboratory Investigation, 39(6), 551–558. https://doi.org/10.3109/00365517909108833

30. Shulman, R. G., & Rothman, D. L. (2001). The "glycogen shunt" in exercising muscle: A role for glycogen in muscle energetics and fatigue. Proceedings of the National Academy of Sciences, 98(2), 457–461. https://doi.org/10.1073/pnas.98.2.457

31. Brooks, G. A. (2020). Lactate as a fulcrum of metabolism. Redox Biology, 35, 101454. https://doi.org/10.1016/j.redox.2020.101454

Chapter 8: Systems, Systems, Systems

32. Robertson, S., & Joyce, D. (2017). Evaluating strategic periodisation in team sport. Journal of Sports Sciences, 36(3), 279–285. https://doi.org/10.1080/02640414.2017.1300315
33. Meeusen, R., Duclos, M., Gleeson, M., Rietjens, G., Steinacker, J. and Urhausen, A. (2006). Prevention, diagnosis and treatment of the Overtraining Syndrome. *European Journal of Sport Science*, 6(1), pp.1–14. doi:10.1080/17461390600617717.

Chapter 9: Be Plastic

34. Colloca, L., & Miller, F. G. (2011). The Nocebo Effect and Its Relevance for Clinical Practice. Psychosomatic Medicine, 73(7), 598–603. https://doi.org/10.1097/psy.0b013e3182294a50

35. Bingel, U., Wanigasekera, V., Wiech, K., Ni Mhuircheartaigh, R., Lee, M. C., Ploner, M., & Tracey, I. (2011). The effect of treatment expectation on drug efficacy: imaging the

analgesic benefit of the opioid remifentanil. Science Transla-
tional Medicine, 3(70), 70ra14. https://doi.org/10.1126/scitra
nslmed.3001244

36. Bartels, J. (2019). Revisiting the Stanford prison experiment,
again: Examining demand characteristics in the guard
orientation. *Journal of Social Psychology*, *159*(6), 780–790.
Retrieved from
https://web.p.ebscohost.com/ehost/detail/detail?vid=28&sid=
94cb0270-a6c9-4691-b5b1-37d97fbe4680%40redis&bdata=Jn
NpdGU9ZWhvc3QtbGl2ZQ%3d%3d#AN=138830635&db=
s3h

37. Crum, A. J., & Langer, E. J. (2007). Mind-Set Matters. Psychological Science, 18(2), 165–171. https://doi.org/10.1111/j.
1467-9280.2007.01867.x

38. How Mental Health Affects Physical Health | Bradley Uni-
versity Online. (2018, June 15). Retrieved from Bradley Univer-
sity Online website: https://onlinedegrees.bradley.edu/blog/h
ow-mental-health-affects- physical-health/

39. Neeper, S. A., et al. Exercise and Brain Neurotrophins. Nature, vol. 373, no. 6510, Jan. 1995, pp. 109–109, 10.1038/373
109a0.

Chapter 10: See More, Do Less

40. Prithishkumar, IJ, and Michael, SA. Understanding Your
Student: Using the VARK Model. Journal of Postgraduate
Medicine, vol. 60, no. 2, 2014, p. 183, 10.4103/0022-3859.132
337.

Chapter 11: What to Do & What Not to Do

-

Chapter 12: Why, Why and a Dash of Why

41. Swann, C., Jackman, P. C., Lawrence, A., Hawkins, R. M., Goddard, S. G., Williamson, O., ... Ekkekakis, P. (2022). The (over)use of SMART goals for physical activity promotion: A narrative review and critique. Health Psychology Review, 1–16. https://doi.org/10.1080/17437199.2021.2023608

42. Kleis, R. R., Hoch, M. C., Hogg-Graham, R., & Hoch, J. M. (2021). The Effectiveness of the Transtheoretical Model to Improve Physical Activity in Healthy Adults: A Systematic Review. Journal of Physical Activity & Health, 18(1), 94–108. Retrieved from https://web.s.ebscohost.com/ehost/pdfviewer/pdfviewer ?vid=8&sid=bd23c06 e-88de-4db3-9d1d-ff3c1bff30f0%40redis

Chapter 13: Back to Basics

-

Chapter 14: Make Your Cake

43. Witard, O. C., Garthe, I., & Phillips, S. M. (2019). Dietary Protein for Training Adaptation and Body Composition Manipulation in Track and Field Athletes. International Journal of Sport Nutrition and Exercise Metabolism, 29(2), 165– 174. https://doi.org/10.1123/ijsnem.2018-0267

44. Roberts, J., Zinchenko, A., Suckling, C., Smith, L., Johnstone, J., & Henselmans, M. (2017). The short-term effect of

high versus moderate protein intake on recovery after strength training in resistance-trained individuals. Journal of the International Society of Sports Nutrition, 14(1). https://doi.org/10 .1186/s12970-017-0201-z

45. Tipton, K. D., Hamilton, D. L., & Gallagher, I. J. (2018). Assessing the Role of Muscle Protein Breakdown in Response to Nutrition and Exercise in Humans. Sports Medicine, 48(1), 53–64. https://doi.org/10.1007/s40279-017-0845-5

46. Wu, G., Fanzo, J., Miller, D. D., Pingali, P., Post, M., Steiner, J. L., & Thalacker- Mercer, A. E. (2014). Production and supply of high-quality food protein for human consumption: sustainability, challenges, and innovations. Annals of the New York Academy of Sciences, 1321(1), 1– 19. https://doi.org/10. 1111/nyas.12500

47. Siri-Tarino, P. W., Sun, Q., Hu, F. B., & Krauss, R. M. (2010). Meta-analysis of prospective cohort studies evaluating the association of saturated fat with cardiovascular disease. The American Journal of Clinical Nutrition, 91(3), 535–546. http s://doi.org/10.3945/ajcn.2009.27725

48. Amirkalali, B., Hosseini, S., Heshmat, R., & Larijani, B. Comparison of Harris Benedict and Mifflin-ST Jeor Equations with Indirect Calorimetry in Evaluating Resting Energy Expenditure. Indian Journal of Medical Sciences, vol. 62, no. 7, 2008, pp. 283–290, www.bioline.org.br/abstract?ms08050.

49. Schroeder, E. C., Franke, W. D., Sharp, R. L., & Lee, D. (2019). Comparative effectiveness of aerobic, resistance, and combined training on cardiovascular disease risk factors: A randomized controlled trial. PLOS ONE, 14(1), e0210292. https: //doi.org/10.1371/journal.pone.0210292

50. Taheri, M., & Arabameri, E. (2012). The effect of sleep deprivation on choice reaction time and anaerobic power of college

student athletes. Asian Journal of Sports Medicine, 3(1), 15–20. Retrieved from https://www.ncbi.nlm.nih.gov/pmc/articles/P MC3307962/

51. Lowrie, J., & Brownlow, H. (2020). The impact of sleep deprivation and alcohol on driving: a comparative study. BMC Public Health, 20(1). https://doi.org/10.1186/s12889-020-09 095-5

52. Rae, D. E., Chin, T., Dikgomo, K., Hill, L., McKune, A. J., Kohn, T. A., & Roden, L. C. (2017). One night of partial sleep deprivation impairs recovery from a single exercise training session. European Journal of Applied Physiology, 117(4), 699–712. https://doi.org/10.1007/s00421-017-3565-5

53. Spiegel, K., Tasali, E., Penev, P., & Cauter, E. V. (2004). Brief Communication: Sleep Curtailment in Healthy Young Men Is Associated with Decreased Leptin Levels, Elevated Ghrelin Levels, and Increased Hunger and Appetite. Annals of Internal Medicine, 141(11), 846. https://doi.org/10.7326/0003-4819-1 41-11-200412070-00008

54. Harding, E. C., Franks, N. P., & Wisden, W. Sleep and thermoregulation. (2020). Current Opinion in Physiology, 15, 7–13. https://doi.org/10.1016/j.cophys.2019.11.008

55. Okamoto-Mizuno, K., & Mizuno, K. (2012). Effects of thermal environment on sleep and circadian rhythm. Journal of Physiological Anthropology, 31(1). https://doi.org/10.1186/1 880-6805-31-14

Chapter 15: Don't Wait Till Monday

Acknowledgements

It's hard to pin down exactly who has contributed to this book as I am the culmination of those around me. Without each and every person, experience, and thought that I have had throughout not just the time writing this book, but the entirety of my life, this book would not be possible. Writing a book is no easy endeavour, I had to employ many of the habits and strategies throughout the book to get to completion. I am not immune to procrastination, stress, or imposter syndrome. So without further dragging, to those around me — family members, friends, editors, past mentors and previous work colleagues, thank you for tolerating, assisting and contributing to the making of this book whether you knew about it or not.

www.ingramcontent.com/pod-product-compliance
Lightning Source LLC
Chambersburg PA
CBHW072058020426
42334CB00017B/1551